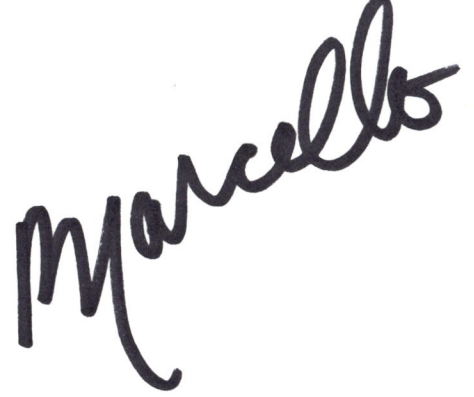

# ONWARDS AND UPWARDS

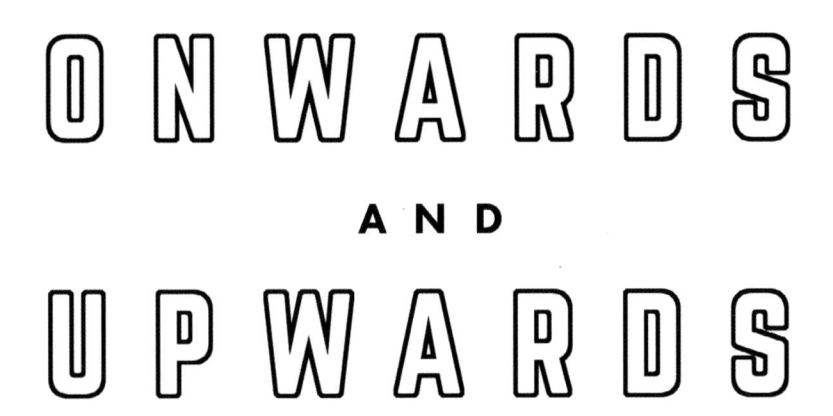

## HOW TO PRIORITIZE YOUR HEALTH AND LIVE YOUR BEST LIFE

MARCELLO PEDALINO

© 2023 Marcello Pedalino

All rights reserved. No part of this publication may be reproduced, distributed, or transmitted in any form or by any means, including photocopying, recording, or other electronic or mechanical methods, without the prior written permission of the publisher, except in the case of brief quotations embodied in critical reviews and certain other non-commercial uses permitted by copyright law.

Print ISBN: 978-1-66789-696-0
eBook ISBN: 978-1-66789-697-7

# TABLE OF CONTENTS

PREFACE ............................................................................... 1

FOREWORD .......................................................................... 3

INTRODUCTION .................................................................... 9

CHAPTER I: TIME ................................................................ 14

CHAPTER II: RECOVERY ..................................................... 18

CHAPTER III: LONGEVITY .................................................. 39

CHAPTER IV: ENERGY ....................................................... 48

CHAPTER V: SLEEP ............................................................ 53

CHAPTER VI: PHYSICAL ENVIRONMENT ......................... 57

CHAPTER VII: INTERPERSONAL ENVIRONMENT ............ 61

CHAPTER VIII: FINANCIAL ENVIRONMENT ..................... 65

CHAPTER IX: EMOTIONAL ENVIRONMENT ..................... 68

EPILOGUE .......................................................................... 70

INSPIRATION ..................................................................... 71

RECOMMENDATION ....................................................... 112

APPRECIATION ................................................................ 113

CONNECTION .................................................................. 114

WORKS CITED .................................................................. 116

ABOUT THE AUTHOR ...................................................... 117

# PREFACE

**I REMEMBER WATCHING PETER JACKSON,** the director of *The Lord of the Rings*, give yet another acceptance speech during the Academy Awards. His epic feature film continued to dominate the evening and smash all box office records. With a large group of cast members and executive producers behind him on stage and several hundred cheering audience members in front of him, Peter finished his notes of gratitude by saying, "Onwards and upwards!" I had never heard that expression before and it resonated deeply. Like the words "Celebrate Life" that came to me while surfing a decade earlier, I adopted this as a new mantra. I knew the minute I heard "Onwards and Upwards" it would make a great title for another book if I were to write one.

Another inspiration for writing this book was my friend from the speaking industry, Alan Berg. While I doubt it would be considered conventional wisdom by most, his passing comment during a business lunch unintentionally touched a competitive nerve in my psyche. Alan, who had already written four books at the time, said something to the effect of, "Yeah, ya know, anybody can write a book… but you really need to have at least two books under your belt if you want to call yourself an author." Ooof. I'm usually pretty good at not taking things personally. I am also well aware that comparison is the thief of joy. That said, despite Alan having no intention of poo-pooing the accomplishment of writing my first book, every now and then I hear something that triggers the Rocky Balboa section of my brain and makes me want to defeat Ivan Drago despite being the underdog and having to train in the snow in Russia.

Anywho, I kinda let it roll off. Kinda, but not really. One of the questions I was often asked at a book signing or speaking engagement while out promoting *Celebrate Life* was "When are you going to write another book?" Now don't get me wrong, writing a book can be a very rewarding and cathartic experience (*it was for me*). However, writing a book is also really freakin' hard. It's tedious.

It's a daunting task. It's an especially daunting task jotting down your stream of consciousness with terrible handwriting on a bunch of random yellow sticky notes and then doing your best to transfer them to an iPad via an extremely inefficient hunt-and-peck method for hours at a time until your butt is sore and your back is stiff.

Alan's comment was akin to what my good friend, Mike Walter, shared with me when I was thirty-six, "The shape you're in at forty is a good indication of the shape you'll be in for the rest of your life." It's not that I was out of shape per se, but man, those words and mindset were (*and still are*) a constant nudge to take care of myself. So, despite never being a great student or listener in school, it tends to resonate when people I admire or respect say something to me, directly or indirectly.

Thank you, Mike, for the reminder to always treat my body with the respect it deserves. Thank you, Alan, for reiterating how important it is to stay humble and stay hungry. And thank you, Peter, for the inspiration to continue moving onwards and upwards.

# FOREWORD

**HOW DO I BEGIN TO** share with you my perspective on the extraordinary man who swept me off my feet and elevated my life beyond my expectations? Well, I'll start by telling you that a person like Marcello Pedalino does not just accidentally pop into your experience. I am a firm believer that we are given what we "ask" for, and even though I may not have been consciously aware of what was coming my way when I met Marcello nearly ten years ago, I knew that I had definitely been asking the Universe to bring me a very particular person, and the Universe did not disappoint.

You and I met at the end of Marcello's first book, *Celebrate Life*, which was less than a year after Marcello and I met. You learned that I am part of a great big Italian family. In fact, I am the eighth of nine children born to two wonderful parents, and I was fortunate enough to enjoy a very happy upbringing filled with an abundance of love and support. Despite my mom's recent passing in 2020 and my oldest sister's passing in 2021, our family, led by my ninety-three-year-old father, has remained strong and deeply connected and is continually growing. In addition to my own family, I am privileged to be a member of the Pedalino family with an equal amount of love and connection. Marcello's dad, Vic, has declared me his favorite daughter-in-law, and even though there are no other daughters-in-law with whom I am competing, I will take it as an honor and a huge compliment. He has even proclaimed that if things didn't work out between Marcello and me, I would be the one who gets to stay in the family! Marcello's mom, Tracy, has been an angel stepping in as "Mom2" since my own mother's transition, and Marcello's sister, Sharmon, is probably the best version of all of them. Family just doesn't get any better.

Marcello and I knew instantaneously that we were a match unlike any of our own previous relationships. I am serious when I say instantaneously—our first date was over a cup of tea that lasted three hours. By the final sip, we both realized that something very special was happening. Amidst the dozens of "coincidences" that took place over the next few months, including finding out that our families are from the same city of Potenza in the south of Italy, the "when is your birthday" conversation finally came up. I was secretly dying to know his sign from the first date, but things were going so incredibly well that I didn't want to mess up our mojo based on my superficial dabblings in astrology and relationship compatibility. When we discovered that our birthdays were only one day apart in February, that moment solidified for us that ours was unlikely a chance meeting and there were greater forces at work here. By the time you finish this book, you, too, will discover that what you choose to focus on, whether you say it out loud or not, ultimately becomes your reality.

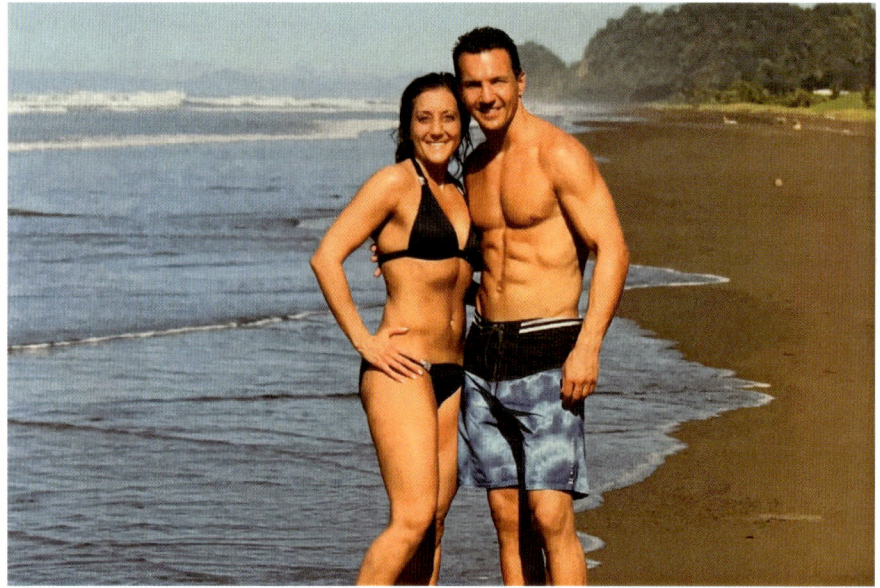

For those of you who remember the last page of *Celebrate Life*, Marcello wrote:

> "She might actually enjoy celebrating life as much as I do and might already have her own admirable version of the 'all in' lifestyle. Together, as a team, the vibrant synergy we produce might be enough to get me to paradise faster than I ever thought possible. And maybe, just maybe…she'll come into my life without any drama or baggage, because that's how 'she rolls.' Nahh… that stuff only happens in the movies. Right?"

I guess Marcello's gut instinct *was* right.

When I was first introduced to Marcello's then-five-year-old daughter, Isabella, I knew that the three of us were going to make an exciting new life for ourselves. Isabella and I bonded very quickly, and a loving relationship began.

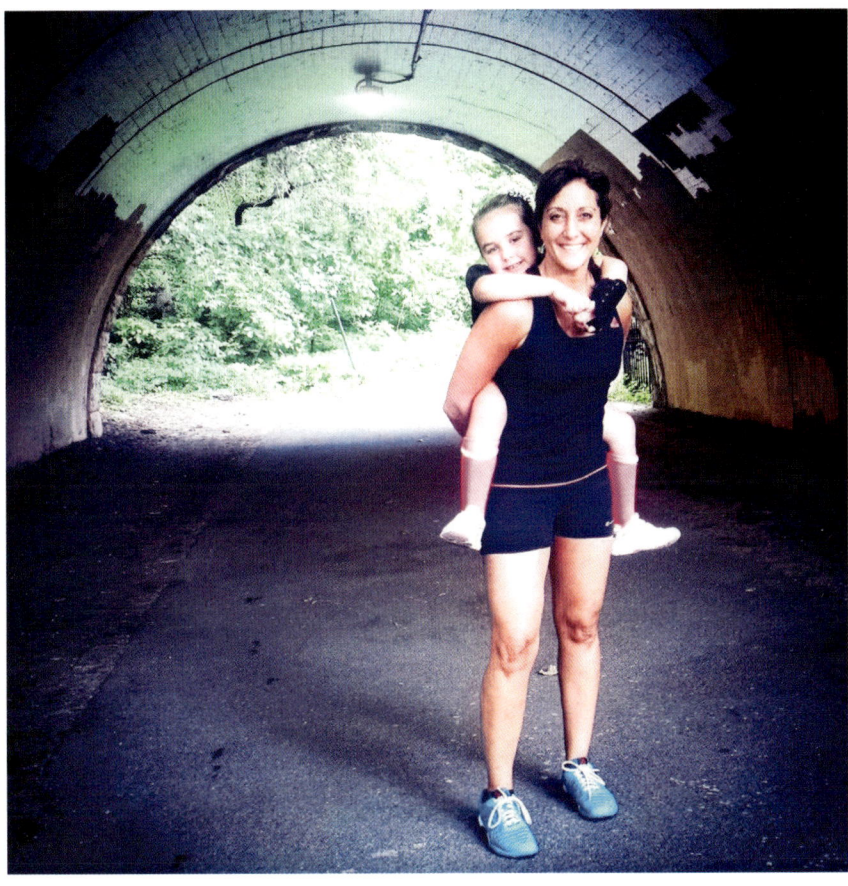

I knew how important it was for me to be a positive influence on Isabella as a strong and capable woman who would always be there for her as a friend, mentor, and shoulder to lean on. I also knew that marrying Marcello meant that I would take on the role of being Isabella's stepmother. Marcello wrote *Celebrate Life* to impart on Isabella the wisdom he learned in his own life, so I knew that I also had to step up to the task. Especially being on the front lines of working with children as a general pediatrician, I knew that she deserved it.

Over the years, I have been a firsthand witness to how Marcello and Isabella have grown in their relationship. I have watched Isabella transition from a small and dependent child into a beautiful and intelligent young lady with the ability to take care of herself and form opinions of her own. I have had the unique opportunity to witness Marcello navigate the predictable but often challenging road of fathering a little girl who, before our eyes, is becoming a young woman. This transition was evident when Isabella tried to put her foot down one day and declared, "I don't have to make my bed today, Daddy. It's a free country!" Although he appreciated the newfound independence that he worked so hard to instill in her, she had her bed made by the time she left for school.

Marcello has remained an incredibly reliable, dependable, and consistently predictable father who encourages Isabella to use her resources, including all he has taught her over the years, to care for her own well-being. Marcello's main mission is to create a world for all three of us in which we are never without, always supported, and always loved. Part of the method to his parenting madness includes putting a dollar into the "Bowl of Honor" for every piece of your laundry that's inside out, having to practice piano before reading for leisure, and making sure to take a few laps around the block after sitting for a while; you just cannot create a self-sufficient and productive adult any other way.

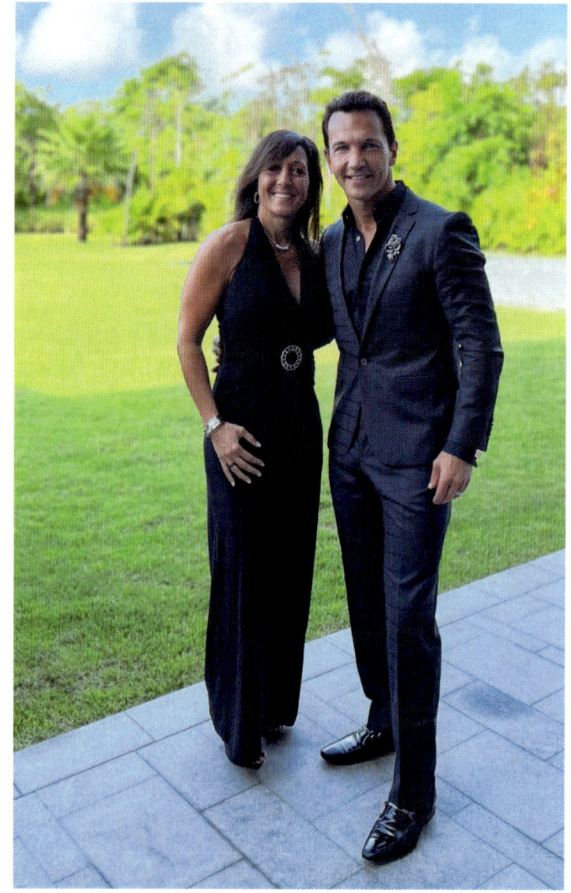

As a husband, Marcello is an openly honest accountability partner. I like the fact that he projects this straight-up, no-frills approach to telling it like it is in his writing as well. I've come to realize that despite Marcello not being traditionally book-smart and never receiving a college degree, his genius lies in the unique, forward-thinking, and sometimes annoying way in which his brain processes information. He is often a step ahead, and he amazes me by seeing the bigger picture when the rest of us are more focused on what is right in front of us. Sometimes his intense and relentless approach is a lot to handle, but I have no doubt that this energy is why he is such a successful entrepreneur. He applies the same passion toward our love affair, making me feel inspired, safe, and encouraged when I wake up next to him each morning. Prior to meeting Marcello, I always appreciated the present while knowing I needed to plan for the next few years. What he has taught me, and as you will read in this book, is that we need to plan for *much* further down the road.

The content of Marcello's first book, *Celebrate Life*, is enough to guide any young person toward a successful future if he or she listens to the recommendations and actually follows them. This second book, *Onwards and Upwards*, takes that foundational knowledge and supercharges it with updated and relevant nuggets of actionable advice. Whether the reader is a young adult looking for some direction on how to be a successful and productive member of society or someone who has already been around the block and wants to either validate their current way of life or make some simple yet meaningful upgrades, *Onwards and Upwards* delivers. Enjoy this book for its simplicity, delight in its brilliant photography, and embrace the wise content that has been compiled as a result of many years of trial and error with incredible growth along the way.

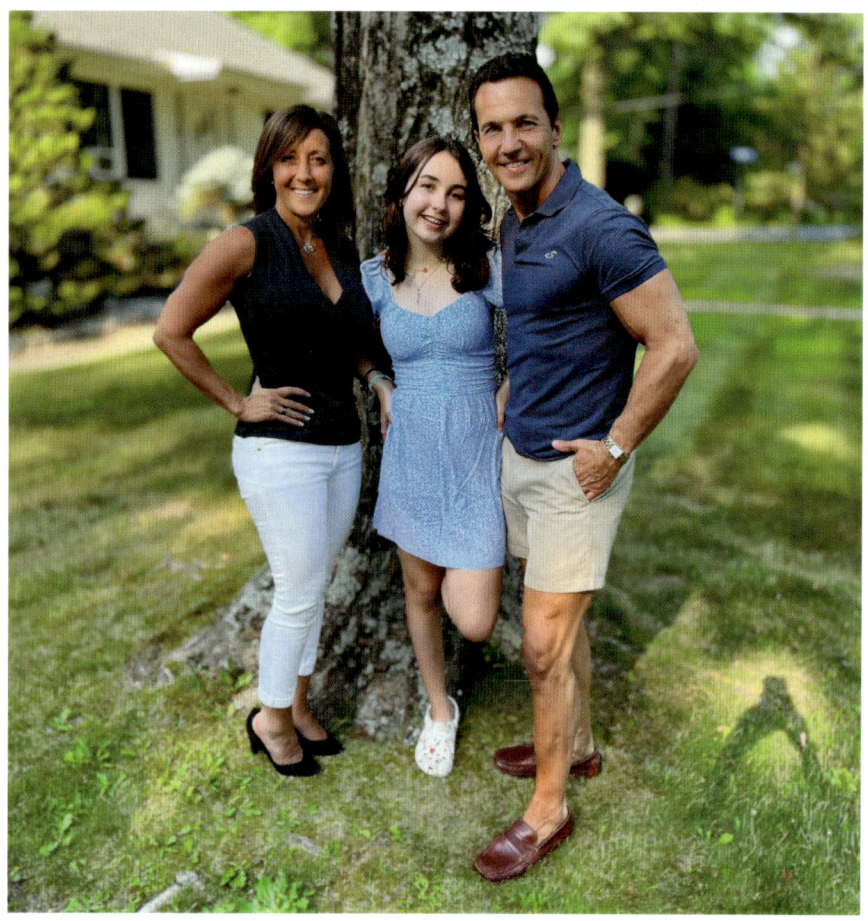

When we met, Marcello and I raised our teacups and christened our new journey by proclaiming, "To the edge!" To this day, we vow to each other that our helmets will always be tightened and our seatbelts always fastened as our toes continually touch the precipice of abundance and opportunity. The edge, to us, is a place where everything is possible, and the *impossible* just takes a little longer. We know that the adventure lies in the journey itself, and we face it without fear of death or pain. So come to the edge with us and let's move onwards and upwards together.

~DR. JILL PEDALINO

# INTRODUCTION

## LET'S GET CAUGHT UP.

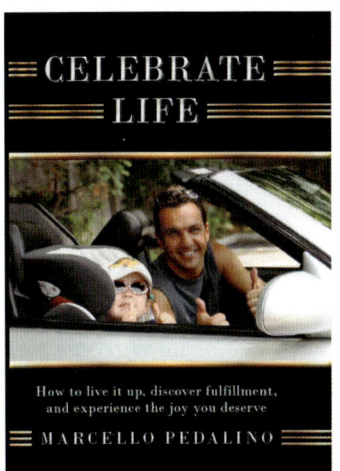

Here's the good news—I'm not dead yet!

When I was writing my first book, *Celebrate Life*, the goal was to teach my then-five-year-old daughter, Isabella, everything I would have ever wanted to teach her about life—just in case I died too soon. I wasn't sick or suffering from anything life-threatening at the time (*at least not in a medical sense*), but I'm a big fan of peace of mind, so I liked knowing that my blueprint for celebrating life would be in Isabella's hands even if I met an untimely death.

More good news: not only am I alive and well, but I've also learned another decade's worth of life lessons and self-care knowledge to fill up another easy-to-read guidebook to pass on to Isabella, to several other people I care about, and to everyone who said they benefitted from reading *Celebrate Life*.

Fortunately, Isabella is a teenager now, and I can share a lot of this new and updated stuff with her in real-time conversations. However, if you have any experience parenting a teenager, you probably know that communicating with one isn't always the easiest thing to do. Admittedly, when I was thirteen years old, I know I wasn't thinking, "Hey, Dad, let's sit down and have a

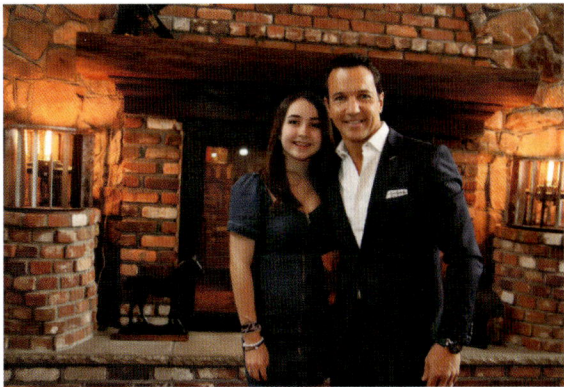

sensible and pragmatic chat for two hours about what could make my life a lot easier when I grow up since you've already gone through most of this crap, and I'm perfectly open to everything you say because you're an adult." Nope. Not even close. As I mentioned in *Celebrate Life*, the quote from Mark Twain still holds true. "The older I get, the smarter my parents get."

Even more good news—the foundation of self-care and the empowerment tips that were featured in *Celebrate Life* still hold up because they are evergreen. The chapters about taking care of yourself, keeping good company, doing what you love, traveling, making a difference, letting things go, and evolving are still meaningful and relevant. Even better? In *Onwards and Upwards,* I share new techniques and concepts in these general areas that have had a very positive impact on both my personal and professional lives that you can implement as well if you want to continue to move onwards and upwards like I did.

I love a good win-win situation. In this case, Isabella gets another book from her dad that will come in handy as she navigates her future, and you get an opportunity to learn some new things (*or light a fire under your butt to start doing something you knew you should've been doing a long time ago*) that can change your life for the better.

Alright. I think that covers the basics. Whether you have read *Celebrate Life* or not, everyone should be caught up now and be literally on the same page. Let's get down to business.

What happened to me isn't important. This book is for YOU. No matter what happened to you, whether it was an injury, crisis, or setback, you can either be a victim or a survivor. In order to survive and advance, endure and conquer, and ultimately move onwards and upwards, you need to prioritize your health. When it comes to living your best life—if you have your health, you have hope. If you have hope, you have everything.

When I wrote *Celebrate Life,* I explained, "How to live it up, discover fulfillment, and experience the joy you deserve"—just like the subtitle promised. The foundation of the book was overall health and wellness. A lot of the positive feedback that I received revolved around my philosophy, "If you can't take care of yourself, you can't take care of the people who depend on you." Basically, if you aren't healthy, nothing else really matters and you're making life way harder than it needs to be. So, in addition to being a big fan of some awesome movie sequels that evolve the storyline and update some important information like *The Empire Strikes Back*, *The Godfather Part Two*, and *Top Gun: Maverick*, I thought you might enjoy another helpful installment of self-care guidance and real talk that could make you a stronger, wiser, and more resilient human in a world that leaves you no choice but to be able to handle ANYTHING that comes your way—even a global pandemic and a polarizing politically charged climate.

In the upcoming pages, I'm going to focus on the importance of sleep hygiene, time-restricted feeding, stress management, strategic muscle development, and longevity. I've learned several new techniques that can help you enjoy meaningful improvements when it comes to your day-to-day readiness status and quality of life as they did for me.

Like last time in *Celebrate Life*, you'll find some little Easter eggs throughout the book.

-

  **MARCELLO'S MESSAGE:**
  If you're like me and sometimes have to read something three times to understand the most important part of the paragraph, I've got you covered. When you see a highlighted section called "Marcello's Message", read the bold print inside because that's some important stuff I don't want you to miss.

-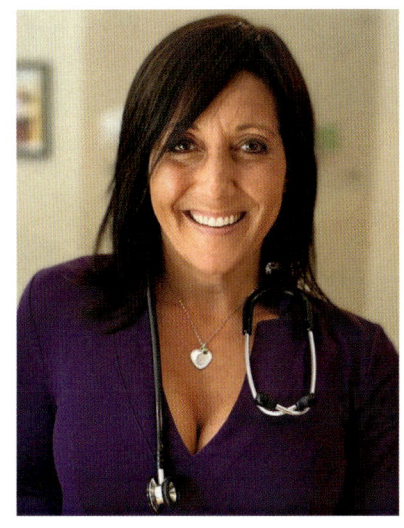

  If you remember the beautiful Italian woman I was standing next to on the beach in the last chapter of *Celebrate Life*, well, I'm happy to report that she became my beautiful wife, and she's a really smart medical physician. Since my education is limited to a couple of basic yet very thorough and helpful certifications in nutrition, fitness, and lifespan, I asked "Dr. Jill" (*as she's affectionately known by all her patients*) to collaborate with me and share her extensive professional medical expertise, scientific data, and female perspective to round out all the research I did.

So, when you read something I wrote followed by a section that says, "Dr. Jill Will See You Now," it's there to drive home the point and give my book a little more "street cred."

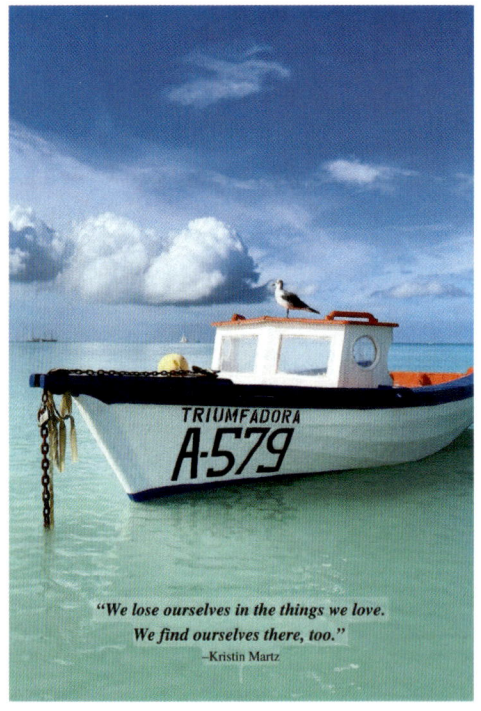

"We lose ourselves in the things we love.
We find ourselves there, too."
–Kristin Martz

- I don't know about you, but I love great quotes that make me think, grow, or remind me about what's really important in life. The same goes for a visually stimulating photo or provocative short story. Throughout the book, you'll see a collection of my photography which, in the end, will be paired with many of my favorite inspirational quotes that I call "Inspo-memes." As someone who is a painfully slow reader, I always appreciate it when I see an enlarged quote, anecdotal short story, or a full-page photo to break up all the text, chapter after chapter.

- Over the years, reading has proven to be a powerful source of inspiration for me both personally and professionally. After the last chapter, you will find a list of book recommendations I've compiled for you with the hope that you will reap the benefits like I did. If you want to read my expanded review of these educational and entertaining books prior to purchasing any of them for your own library, check out all of the "Marcello Recommends" articles on my blog over at MarcelloPedalino.com.

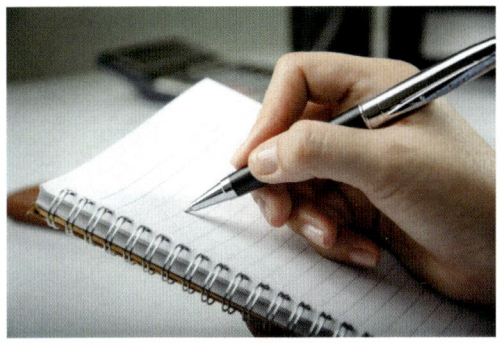

And finally, even though I never liked it when I was given homework in school, I strategically placed a few thought-provoking questions throughout the book that will require some extra effort on your end so you can be an active participant and maximize the benefits of this reading experience. The questions are designed for you to identify areas of your life that may need your immediate attention. By the time you finish the last chapter, you'll be able to review the answers, develop a game plan, and take that first step toward moving onwards and upwards.

Ok, I think that covers everything. Let's do this.

## CHAPTER 1:

# TIME

There was a businessman from New York City. You know the type—he's got the Rolex, sports car, and a summer home in the Hamptons. He went to his doctor for his annual checkup and the doctor said, "Look, pal, you're only fifty years old and couldn't even walk up the stairs to my office without being out of breath. You're stressed out, overweight, and sleep-deprived. If you don't make some changes and take a vacation real soon, you're not going to make it back here for next year's appointment."

The businessman took his doctor's advice and booked a trip to Mexico at a nice little all-inclusive resort. Unfortunately, on the first night of his vacation, he got an emergency call from the office. A big deal that he had been working on had gone south, and they needed him to make a bunch of calls and sit in on some zoom meetings so he could clean up the mess. He took care of everything as usual. But now, he couldn't get back to sleep. So around five o'clock in the morning he finally said to himself, "I might as well go for a walk on the beach."

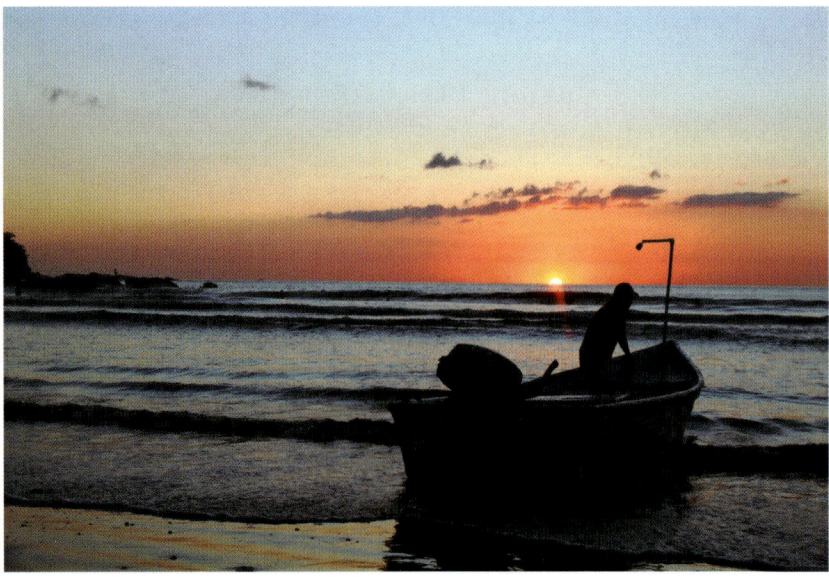

As the sun was coming up, the businessman saw a little fishing boat with three big beautiful yellowfin tuna inside. Then he saw the fisherman walking back down to his boat. He was in his thirties, fit, tan, and smiling from ear to ear. The businessman said, "Wow, that's a very impressive catch! Are you going back out for more?"

"No, señor, I have enough. This is enough to pay my bills and feed my family."

The businessman said, "Really? What are you going to do for the rest of the day?"

The fisherman replied, "Well, I'll go play with my kids, then make love to my wife, take a siesta, have a nice family dinner, then go out to see my friends, listen to some music, and have a few laughs."

The businessman couldn't believe it. He said, "Listen, pal, I've got an MBA from Harvard. I can help you get this little fishing operation of yours to the next level. First, you're going to start fishing twice a day. You'll catch twice as many fish and make twice as much money."

"And then what, señor?"

"Then you can hire another guy, get another boat, and then cut out the middleman so you can sell your fish directly to the customer. Then you can hire more guys, get more boats, catch more fish, make more money, and go buy a warehouse over in Mexico City."

"And then what, señor?"

"Then you'll be making enough money to open up your own tuna fish cannery in Los Angeles and then finally move your national headquarters to New York City where you can take the company public, offer an IPO, and make millions and millions of dollars!"

"Wow, señor. How long will all that take?"

Without missing a beat, the businessman said, "fifteen, twenty, twenty-five years... TOPS! And then you can retire!!!"

"And then what, señor?"

"Then you can finally spend some time at your home in Mexico, fish a little in the morning, play with your kids, make love to your wife, take a siesta, have dinner with your family, then go out with your friends, listen to some music...and have a few laughs."

The fisherman smiled politely, shook his head, and said, "No gracias, señor. No thank you, have a nice day."

**I'D LIKE TO THANK** my good friend, Jorge Lopez, for sharing the story of The Mexican Fisherman with me many years ago and Heinrich Bolls, the original author of *The Mexican Fisherman* story. It had a profound impact on my lifestyle choices and business model.

Look, there's nothing wrong with growing your business and making a lot of money. Trust me, I get it—I'm a capitalist at heart. I just want you to appreciate that success comes with a price ...and the currency is time.

**MARCELLO'S MESSAGE:**
*SUCCESS COMES WITH A PRICE...AND THE CURRENCY IS TIME.*

I promised myself that I would continue to pay it forward like Jorge did and share this story whenever the opportunity presented itself. I knew when it was time for my second book, it needed to be included. After sharing my version of *The Mexican Fisherman* with audiences during several opening keynote speaking presentations since writing *Celebrate Life*, it seemed like a perfect way to kick off this book.

Where do you see *yourself* fifteen, twenty, twenty-five years from now? What does it look like? What do YOU look like? Regardless of the magnitude of your goals, whether you want to take your company public and make millions and millions of dollars, or find something you love to do and make just enough to support your family and enjoy the simple things in life, at some point you're going to have to do some serious introspection and a personal lifestyle evaluation. This critical process will include reevaluating the amount of time you are spending with people or things that don't support the vision your heart and gut are guiding you toward. The bottom line is that the sooner you realize what truly brings you joy in life, the sooner you can start to budget your time accordingly.

**MARCELLO'S MESSAGE:**
*THE SOONER YOU REALIZE WHAT TRULY BRINGS YOU JOY IN LIFE, THE SOONER YOU CAN START TO BUDGET YOUR TIME ACCORDINGLY.*

Time is truly a priceless commodity, especially when it is time spent with your family. There will always be people, things, and life itself that will try to get in the way of you spending time with your parents and kids. (*Some by chance, some on purpose.*) Do the best you can, as often as you can, with what you've got to work with—and make it happen. At some point in your life, you (*and your family members*) will realize that making the effort was worth it beyond measure.

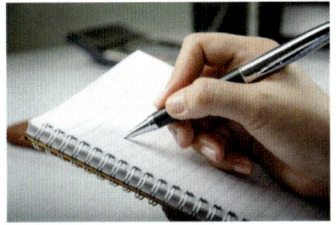

- Do you aspire to be more like the Mexican fisherman or the businessman from New York City? Why?

  _____

  _____

  _____

- Who or what is worth your time, effort, and energy?

  _____

  _____

  _____

## CHAPTER II:
# RECOVERY

**ONCE YOU'VE SYNCHRONIZED YOUR TIME** to match your life goals, you will need to appreciate the importance of recovery along your journey. Regardless of your lifestyle choice, you can only maintain a sustainable pace by successfully managing the inevitable bumps and bruises that will occur as you navigate your path.

If we are being honest with ourselves, I think we can agree that most of us are recovering from something. Perhaps it was an illness, injury, death of a loved one, divorce or break up, financial crisis, business setback, natural disaster, or even a freakin' global pandemic! Unless you've been living in a plastic bubble, you're either trying to recover from something right now or you will eventually need to recover from some of the hardest days and/or years of your life. The sheer fact that you still have a pulse after all the recent craziness in our world is a true testament to your hustle, grit, and, yeah, probably some luck sprinkled in. So, kudos to you!

Now what?

Let's focus on some of the things that you should and shouldn't be doing from this day forward to continue to move onwards and upwards. You might know that my wife and I are pretty dialed in when it comes to nutrition, sleep, and exercise. However, the fourth element that not everyone appreciates and most people underestimate is the power of stress reduction and how important it is for recovery. I hear people say all the time that they want "work-life balance." Well, that's never going to happen if your stress levels are through the roof because it's a fact that tension obliterates balance.

**MARCELLO'S MESSAGE:**
*TENSION OBLITERATES BALANCE.*

## DR. JILL WILL SEE YOU NOW

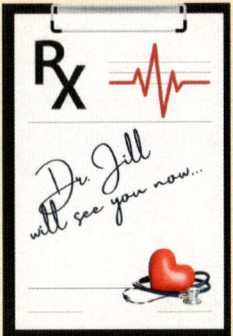

*Stress is more toxic than we may think. It can, and I promise you it will, sabotage any diet or workout plan you are trying to maintain. We've all heard of the fight-or-flight response to stress, and this amazing and very healthy mechanism has been a driving force to allow humans to survive over the millions of years of our evolution. Our brain switches on the fight-or-flight response whenever it thinks we are in danger. It does this by thinking that it if can help us run from danger, or fight against it, it will help us to survive. These days, our stressors are no longer running from a saber-tooth tiger, but rather job loss, financial woes, and relationship issues, to name a few. The problem is that the brain doesn't differentiate between a physical threat and an emotional threat, so, regardless of the trigger, a very sophisticated cascade of enzymatic chain reactions ensues, causing cortisol and adrenaline to rise, the immune system to become suppressed, and a host of other changes like increased blood sugar, digestion problems, and cardiovascular strain increasing the risk of heart attack and stroke. Current statistics state that upwards of eighty-four percent of Americans report feeling stressed weekly, and it is estimated that over seventy percent of many Americans' day is spent in fight-or-flight mode. Those are some frightening numbers and a sobering reminder that we must start taking back control of our stress responses.*

*Despite the fast-paced and very stress-inducing modern life we are living, all hope is not lost. Something as simple as laughter strengthens the immune system, boosts mood, diminishes pain, and protects us from the damaging effects of stress. Nothing works faster or more dependably to bring our mind and body back into balance than a good laugh. Like a cleansing deep breath, a laugh is free, and you can always pull it out of your bag of tricks wherever you are.*

One of the most powerful stress reduction tools I've learned in the past decade was appreciating the power of the word "good."

At the time when I wrote *Celebrate Life*, the best tool that I had was tuning in to the fictional radio station, WKIP (We Keep It Positive). Throughout my twenty-year friendship with my buddy Mike, he and I have done our best to see the bright side of things regardless of how dark they get. The idea is that by dialing into the right frequency, you have the ability to make the best of any situation.

Since then, I have discovered Jocko Willink, the well-known American author and retired U.S. Navy SEAL, and I really gravitated toward his way of thinking. Jocko takes the stoic philosophy of nothing in life being inherently "good" or "bad," but merely whatever we make it one step further by declaring that *everything* is good. He says,

> "Mission got canceled? Good. You can focus on another one. Got tapped out? Got beat? Good. You learned. Unexpected problems? Good. You have the opportunity to figure out a solution. When things are going bad, don't get all bummed out, don't get startled, don't get frustrated. If you can say the word 'good,' guess what? It means you're still alive. You're still breathing. And if you're still breathing, you still have some fight left in you. So, get up, dust off, reload, recalibrate, reengage, and go out on the attack."

Right on! Jocko definitely nails it when putting stress into perspective. Now, let's practice some real-world examples:

- Your best and most valuable employee gives notice at a very inconvenient time for your business. What are you going to say? "Good." Everyone is replaceable and you will find someone better. As Mike always says, "Talent moves on. Get over it."

- You are personally trying to work a full-time job, care for an ailing family member, and get your kids to every one of their after-school activities, all while volunteering out of guilt for something to which you knew you didn't have the time nor energy to commit, so you end up in the hospital with a bleeding ulcer. What are you going to say? "Good." Now you will appreciate the brilliant wisdom and advice of my business-savvy colleague, Jeffrey Craig Siber: "Delegate or suffocate." The sooner you realize that you can't be in two places at once and that there will be times when you need to ask for help (*no matter how independent you are*), the sooner you'll be able to harness the power of strategic collaboration. Further, if you are an entrepreneur and/or a parent, there are times when you'll need to accept, like I did, the reality of the concept, "It's not my fault, but it is my problem." No matter how much you prepare or how flawless your own execution is, there will be a client, team member, or child whose actions will require you to expend additional time and energy to rectify the situation.

When coping with stress, it is important to acknowledge the relationship between stress and fear. The interesting thing about stress is that it's usually based on fear and being afraid of what *might* go wrong in the future. So, the reality is that fear lives in the future, and since I think we can all agree that the future doesn't exist yet, consider this: if fear lives in the future, and the future doesn't exist, then fear doesn't exist.

**MARCELLO'S MESSAGE:**
*IF FEAR LIVES IN THE FUTURE, AND THE FUTURE DOESN'T EXIST, THEN FEAR DOESN'T EXIST.*

By the way, most of the things we worry about never happen, anyway. It's a waste of energy. But, let's keep it real and be pragmatic. Of course, you should always have a plan, a backup plan, and a backup plan to the backup plan when it comes to something really important. However, the futility of burning through valuable emotional energy reserves by stressing out unnecessarily was validated by a great family man and entrepreneur, Ben Stowe. I interviewed him a few years back and asked him, "What's something you need to spend less time doing?" He replied, "I need to spend less time worrying because it's always the things you don't see comin' that get ya anyway."

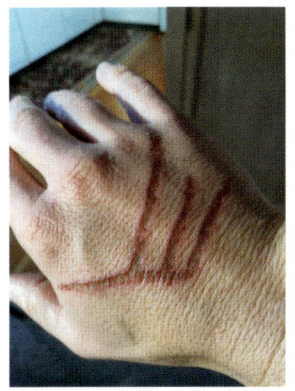

I couldn't agree more, Ben.

This photo shows the very unexpected result of focusing so much on unclogging our bathroom sink that I accidentally spilled a few drops of caustic liquid drain cleaner on my hand, causing a third-degree burn and permanent scarring. When people ask me about this very noticeable disfiguration of the back of my hand, I share the true story, but I secretly wish it was something cooler and more heroic, like fighting off a shark attack or rescuing a baby from a burning house.

Now, take a look at this cool little story about perspective.

## GOOD THING, BAD THING:

*There was once a farmer who owned a horse and had a son. One day, his horse ran away. The neighbors came to express their concerns. "Oh, that's too bad. How are you going to work the fields now?"*

*The farmer replied, "Good thing, bad thing, who knows?"*

*In a few days, his horse came back and brought another horse with her. Now, the neighbors were glad. "Oh, how lucky! Now you can do twice as much work as before!"*

*The farmer replied, "Good thing, bad thing, who knows?"*

*The next day, the farmer's son fell off the new horse and broke his leg. The neighbors were concerned again. "Now that he is incapacitated, your son can't help you around; that's too bad."*

*The farmer replied, "Good thing, bad thing, who knows?"*

*Soon, the news came that a war had broken out, and all the young men were required to join the army. The villagers were sad because they knew that many of the young men would not come back. The farmer's son could not be drafted because of his broken leg. His neighbors were envious. "How lucky! You get to keep your only son."*

*The farmer replied, "Good thing, bad thing, who knows?"*

The important thing to remember here is that in order to achieve this coveted position of being able to say the word "good," *no matter how bad things get*, your mental toughness reserves need to be kept as high as possible at all times. How do you do that? You consistently do things that make you happy and reduce your stress. I've got friends who do everything from jiu-jitsu to yoga to gardening to biking to walking their dog to playing an instrument to chilling out.

**MARCELLO'S MESSAGE:**
IN ORDER TO ACHIEVE THIS COVETED POSITION OF BEING ABLE TO SAY THE WORD, "GOOD," NO MATTER HOW BAD THINGS GET, YOUR MENTAL TOUGHNESS RESERVES NEED TO BE KEPT AS HIGH AS POSSIBLE AT ALL TIMES.

ONWARDS AND UPWARDS

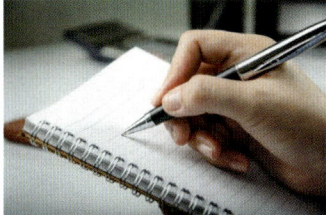

- Which activities make you happy or reduce your stress levels?

_____
_____
_____

_____

Once you've identified activities that make you happy and reduce your stress levels, life starts to get way less complicated. It's actually an embarrassingly simple formula. If something feels good, do it some more. Then, make it a habit and schedule time to do it every day or a few times each week.

For example, even though she hasn't yet gotten the lead role in a theater production or the big solo in one of her choir concerts, Isabella continues to show up and enthusiastically participate at every rehearsal and performance even if she only gets the part of Dopey's understudy in *Snow White and the Seven Dwarfs*, or "Pig #3" in the musical, *Shrek*. The feeling of camaraderie and community fuels her personal sense of joy and the rush of endorphins that comes from singing and dancing on stage should not be underestimated.

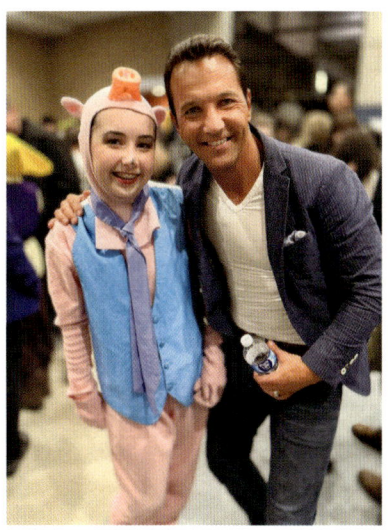

### DR. JILL WILL SEE YOU NOW

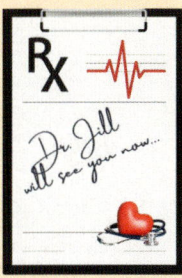

There's no one right answer to what to do when it comes to reducing stress. Many of you are already aware of how meditation and gratitude practices help manage stress. As I mentioned earlier, even something simple as taking a few deep breaths during the day helps with stress, but you may not be aware of the connection between managing your gut microbiome and stress. Our gut is our largest immune organ after our skin. Our intestines are lined with a jelly-like layer of bacteria (as well as viruses and yeast) called the brush border. Think of this layer as a garden made of trillions of bacterial cells that work with our immune system to keep our bodies functioning optimally. If we feed that garden too much sugar and processed foods from our diet, we will create "weeds" instead of "flowers" and we will promote the growth of bacterial species that research has shown actually leads to weight gain and disease.

Did you also know that seventy percent of our body's serotonin (the feel-good hormone) is made by our gut bacteria? Scientists used to think it was made only in the brain, but it's made in the gut, too. We've all heard about the brain-gut connection (like butterflies in your stomach before you do something that you are nervous about). Well, this is partly why. Feeling depressed and anxious often leads to eating foods high in sugar, which feels good—at the moment. Our early ancestors didn't have access to much sugar, so eating sugar activated the pleasure centers of the brain to help them look for more. These days, sugary foods are available everywhere and all the time. Eating sugary foods speeds up that vicious cycle of emotional eating and allows more weeds to grow in that garden. Eating healthier will increase the specific bacteria that create serotonin, which can make us happier. When we feel happier, more motivated, and more in control of our lives, we will naturally want to eat better. This will promote more good bacteria, which will create more serotonin, and the cycle will spiral upward instead of downward. Please trust that our bodies are highly intelligent and resilient organisms capable of incredible recovery if we just give them the opportunity to do so. Positive momentum is what speeds up recovery and increases longevity.

Marcello will take a deeper dive into longevity in the next chapter, but first, check out some of his personal stress-reduction tips.

If you're like me and really appreciate actionable advice that is neatly spelled out for you, you'll love these next couple of pages. The content is designed for those of you who want to take steps in the right direction toward a specific goal, but don't know where to begin or what to expect along the way. The following items should help you go out and start making things happen to reduce your stress levels as soon as you finish reading this chapter.

- **TAKE A WALK:** As long as it's not too dark or icy on the sidewalk or trail, just lace up your sneakers and get movin'. (*Over the past ten* *years, I've seen a ton of people wearing crocs and slip-on flip flops as part of their everyday wardrobe. They might be great for comfort and working virtually from home, but you definitely want proper ankle support and a secure fit when you head outside.)* Walking is simple and it's free. No fancy Peloton or other expensive piece of equipment is necessary. Start with a leisurely yet purposeful stroll for ten minutes your first time out. Then, build yourself up to thirty minutes by increasing your time by a few minutes each week. Try to walk three to five times per week. Bonus: If the sun is out, put on a little sunscreen and reap all the benefits that come with exposure to Vitamin D. Double bonus: There is an actual practice called "Nature Bathing" based on Shinrin Yoku (Forest Bathing), a Japanese practice from the 1950s. Simply spending twenty minutes intentionally interacting with the great outdoors can boost mood and attitude and have a ripple effect on your entire day.

- **VOLUNTEER:**

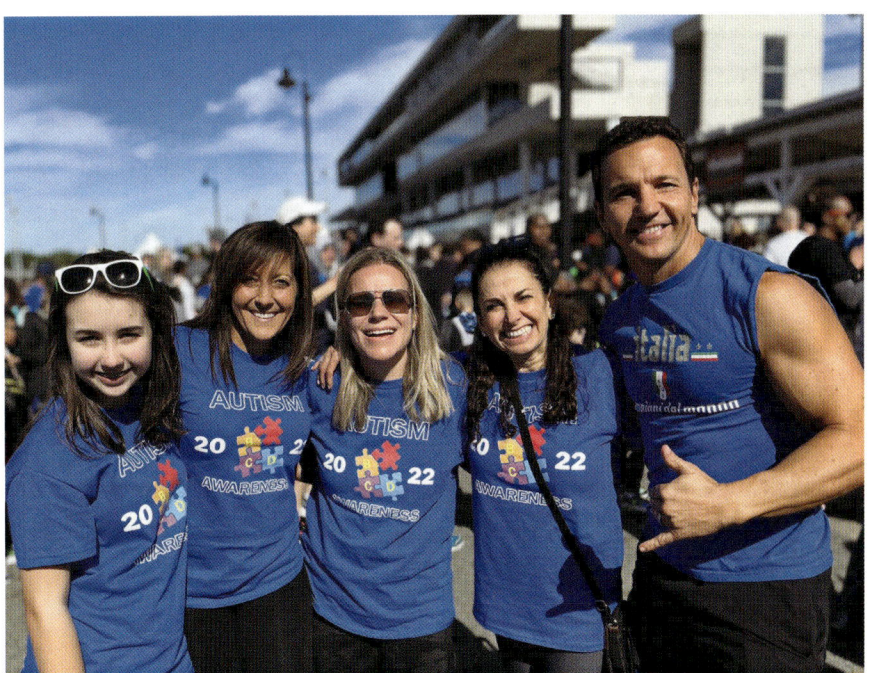

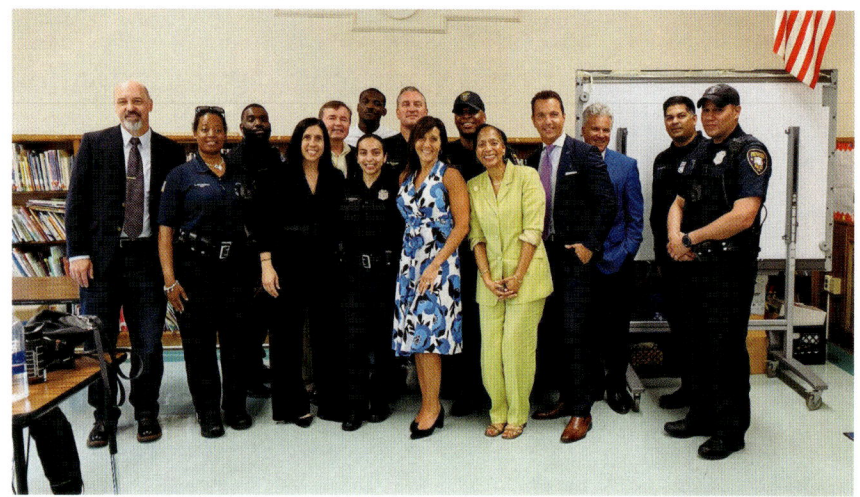

One of my mantras is Do Good, Feel Good. One of the best ways to feel good about yourself and get the serotonin flowing is to do something nice for someone else. In *Celebrate Life*, there was a chapter called "Make a Difference." The only thing that changed is that we found some additional noteworthy organizations that you can support. If you can't find any local organizations to help out, here are a few of our favorites: Covenant House, Habitat for Humanity, Wounded Warrior Project, Tunnel to Towers Foundation, Autism Speaks, Larimer Humane Society, Never Alone Again Resource Center, Kindness for Christopher, Distributing Dignity, and Juvenile Diabetes Research Fund (JDRF).

- **REDISCOVER SOMETHING YOU ENJOY DOING:** Stir up some feel-good nostalgia and pick up an old favorite pastime of yours. Maybe it was chess, hiking, poetry, stamp collecting, crossword puzzles, reading, knitting, remote control cars, photography, or arts and crafts. Or maybe it's time to expand your horizons. Check out your local paper or online bulletin board and see what's happening in your area. It's usually pretty easy to find some fun meetings or clubs that are open to new members. Oftentimes they are free to join or only charge a minimal fee to keep the lights on. There's a good chance you'll be introduced to some potential new hobbies or, more importantly, new friends.

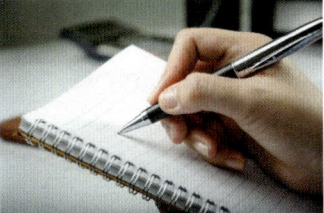

- Write down an old hobby or extracurricular activity that you used to love to do and/or something new that you want to try.

_____

_____

_____

- **SHUT UP AND DANCE:** Take some advice from the 2014 hit song by Walk the Moon. Even if you're in your underwear in the house by yourself like Tom Cruise in *Risky Business*, crank up the volume on your Alexa or Spotify playlist and have at it! (*Pro Tip: Your teenage daughter might really love Broadway musicals so there's a good chance you'll need to endure campy show tune soundtracks on repeat quite often. \*Noise cancelling AirPods can work wonders.*)

- **FOCUS ON WHAT YOU CAN CONTROL:** The best way to stress yourself out is to perseverate over things outside your control like the weather, a traffic jam, peace in the Middle East, how high your taxes are, and people who are committed to Face-Timing a friend as loud as they can in public on speakerphone. Instead, use your energy to think of something productive you will do when this challenging episode is over, or just simply take ten deep breaths and remind yourself how fortunate you were to wake up breathing this morning.

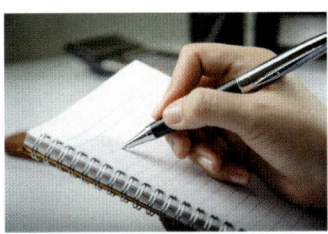

- Is there an aspect of your life that you need to stop trying to control?

_____

_____

_____

- **WAKE UP EARLIER:** Chapter five takes a deeper dive into the importance of good sleep hygiene, but for now just focus on waking up thirty minutes earlier. (*Mike and I are still very proud to emulate the old commercial for the U.S. Marines Corps and say that "We can get more done by 9 a.m. than most people can get done all day."*) You'll be amazed by how much more productive you can be. When you get stuff done and head into your day with positive momentum versus trying to start from behind the eight ball because you're running late and your mind is trying to play catch up, your stress levels have no choice but to improve. (*This will not work if you spend these thirty minutes on your phone doing a FOMO session on social media.*) Keep in mind, you'll probably need to go to bed thirty minutes sooner to help even out your circadian rhythm. Before you start complaining that you're too busy after work, after studying, or after putting the kids to bed, take a hard look at what you normally do before bedtime each night throughout the week. When I do lifestyle audits for clients, nine out of ten times I find upwards of six hours per week are wasted binge-watching something on Netflix or mindlessly scrolling through Tik Tok videos.

- **CREATE A MANTRA AND REPEAT IT:**

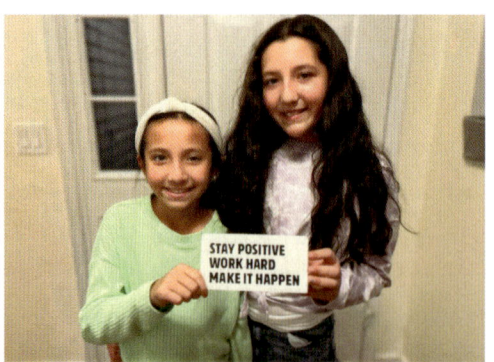

Jill's sister, Tracey, and her husband, Roland, understand the importance of creating a positive atmosphere for their children and themselves. I love walking into their home and having my nieces, Zoey and Macy, show me their family's mantra and how their mom and dad make it easy to remember each day.

Our whole family is big on positive self-talk. (*More on this concept and some potentially life-changing Buddha mojo in the last chapter.*)

Studies have shown that self-soothing techniques like reciting affirmations and praying can do wonders to help individuals chill and reset when the need arises. If you ever watched the character Stuart Smalley on *Saturday Night Live* in the '90s, you might picture someone holding up a mirror in front of their face and saying, "I'm good enough, I'm smart enough, and gosh darn it—people like me." It was a funny comedy bit, and although it was an exaggeration of someone practicing affirmations, at its core, the sketch was indirectly promoting an extremely powerful self-care tool, and Stuart was definitely on to something. You can skip the part about worrying whether people like you since, most of the time, that's irrelevant, but knowing that you are "enough" more often than not is a potent stress reducer. This is especially true in an age where "enough" is determined (*inaccurately*) by the number of views or likes your posts get on social media. Jill and I have a few mantras and affirmations that provide a source of constant empowerment, like "Good begets good, begets good, begets good." It's the idea that you are what you think. Do you want more good stuff to happen? Spend more of your time thinking about what to do if things go *right* versus what to do if things go *wrong*. Feel free to copy a mantra if you can't think of something. I love Sylvester Stallone and his Rocky films. (*The first four, anyway.*) This gem actually came from Rocky V, when Rocky was giving his bratty son a little reality check:

> "Let me tell you something you already know. The world ain't all sunshine and rainbows. It's a very mean and nasty place, and I don't care how tough you are it will beat you to your knees and keep you there permanently if you let it. You, me, or nobody is gonna hit as hard as life. But it ain't about how hard ya hit. It's about how hard you can get hit and keep moving forward. How much you can take and keep moving forward. That's how winning is done! Now if you know what you're

> worth, then go out and get what you're worth. But you gotta be willing to take the hits, and not pointing fingers saying you ain't where you wanna be because of him, or her, or anybody! Cowards do that and that ain't you! You're better than that!"

Isabella has her own mantra that we refer to often. If she gets sick, has a challenging interaction with some mean girls at school, or is about to go up a big hill on her bike, she will say this to herself or out loud:

### THE ISABELLA CREED:

I believe in myself.
I'm strong, smart, beautiful, and kind.
I make things happen.
I keep movin' forward.
I don't quit. I don't lie.
No excuses.
I know that I'm the product of my thoughts.
I know that the Universe is listening.
Pura Vida.
Hakuna Matata.
Celebrate Life.
That's how winnin' is done.
That's how I roll.
Let's do this.

We added in the part about lying when my daily question, "Did you brush your teeth and put on deodorant?" was getting a cranky "Yes, Daddy" response, but wasn't always gettin' done. Yes, I channeled some of my dad's law enforcement investigative techniques by checking if the clear Scotch tape seal that I put over the toothpaste cap was broken after my initial interrogation took place. If you hadn't already guessed, it was not. It was fun to be right, but it proved that she, in fact, did not brush her teeth. I don't think any parent likes to get lied to by anyone, I know I sure don't, but there is some satisfaction that comes from standing your ground and getting to the truth.

Speaking of lying, I've learned over the years that adults lie just as freely and as often as kids do. Dr. Jill recently shared this story with me. I thought you'd enjoy it and have a good laugh the next time you have to try and outsmart your teenager or employee.

### THE SUGAR BOWL:

*An Italian mother, Mrs. Ravioli, came to visit her son, Anthony, for dinner. He lived with a female roommate, Maria. During the course of the meal, his mother couldn't help but notice how pretty Anthony's roommate was. She had long been suspicious of a relationship between the two, and this had only made her more curious. Over the course of the evening, while watching the two interact, she started to wonder if there was more between Anthony and his roommate than met the eye. Reading his mom's thoughts, Anthony volunteered, "I know what you must be thinking, but I assure you, Maria and I are just roommates."*

*About a week later, Maria came to Anthony, saying, "Ever since your mother came to dinner, I've been unable to find the silver sugar bowl. You don't suppose she took it, do you?"*

*"Well, I doubt it, but I'll email her just to be sure." So, he sat down and wrote an email.*

*Dear Mama,*

*I'm not saying that you "did" take the sugar bowl from my house; I'm not saying that you "did not" take it. But the fact remains that it has been missing ever since you were here for dinner.*

*Love, Anthony*

*Several days later, Anthony received an email response from his mama, which read,*

Dear Son,

*I'm not saying that you "do" sleep with Maria; I'm not saying that you "do not" sleep with her. But the fact remains that if she were sleeping in her OWN bed, she would have found the sugar bowl by now.*

Love, Mama

- **PLAN A VACATION:** (*and have it written down on your calendar*)
  It's not just the trip itself; it's the lead-up time before the trip. Getting through a tough couple of months or even years will still be tough, but knowing that there is a light at the end of the tunnel by having a date written down on your calendar is an incredible stress-reduction hack.

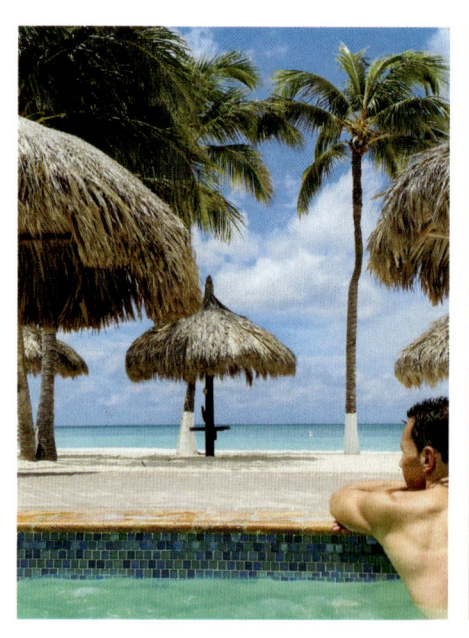

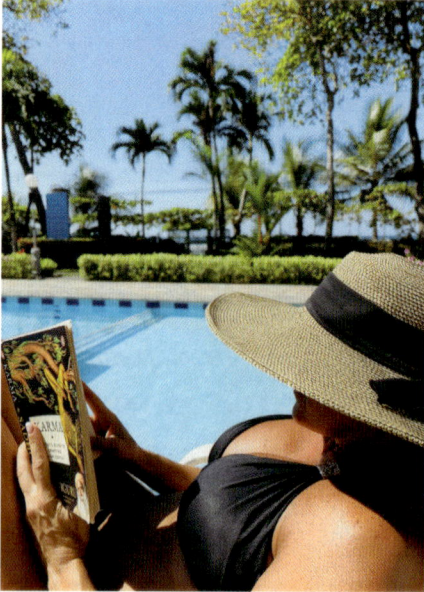

We happen to be big fans of the beach, so Aruba and Costa Rica are our favorite oasis go-to destinations. (*I'm pretty sure that I've got some sort of seasonal affective disorder that limits my sanity and will-power during the winter months here in Jersey. I'm all good for Spring, Summer, and Fall. Once January hits, my need to see and feel the sunshine reaches DEFCON 4.*) If, by chance, you also enjoy the beach, mountains, and some really nice people, Dr. Jill and I have a place in Costa Rica that we rent out. Visit CelebrateLifeCondo.com for more details and to make reservations.

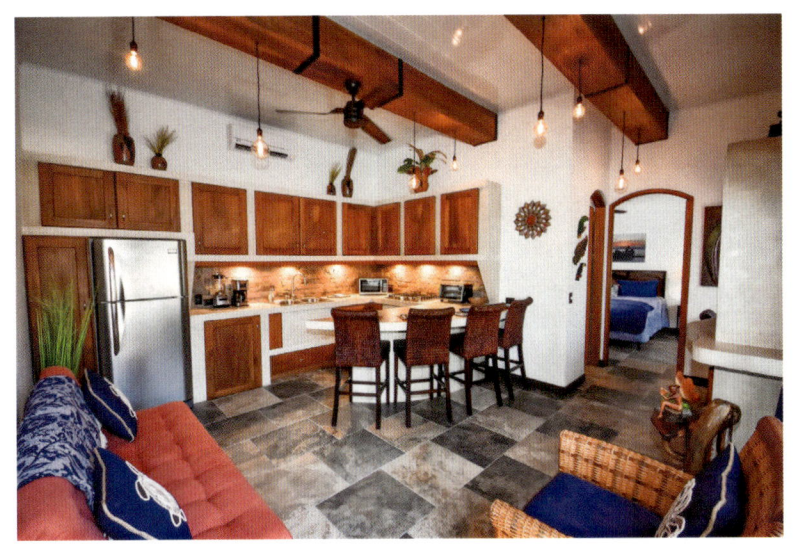

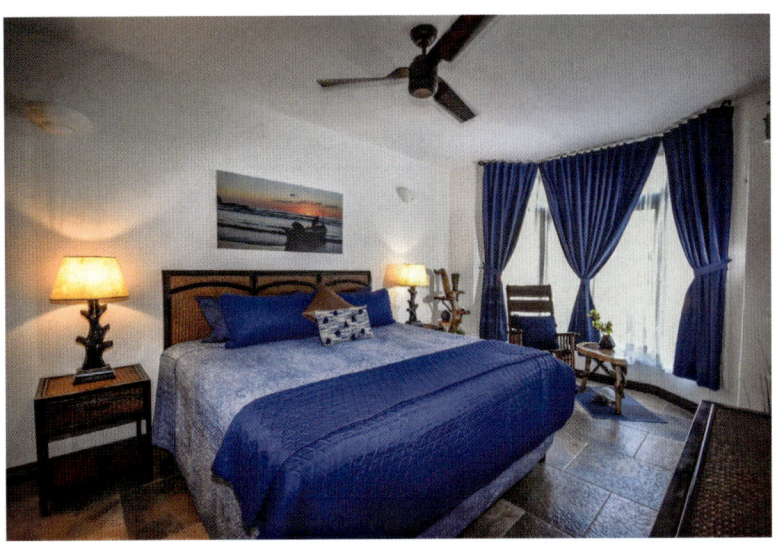

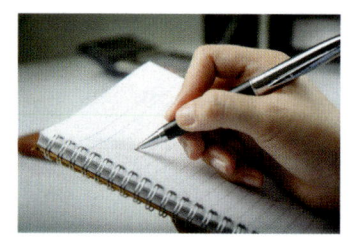

- Is there a travel destination on your bucket list?

  _____
  _____
  _____

- **TURN OFF THE NEWS AND WATCH A MOVIE INSTEAD:** I don't normally recommend sitting down on the couch for two hours, but if you can watch a movie that might inspire you to persevere, exemplify how to be a better person, or make you laugh out loud, I'm all for it. Besides, if you haven't noticed, most news programs are filled with death, destruction, divisiveness, and despair. (*And in most cases, there's nothing you can do about it, so it's like inviting Mike Tyson to punch you in the face three times and then sticking around so he can do it again and again. Yeah, I know it seems like an extreme example, but that's what watching the news is really like.*) I used to think that "If it bleeds, it leads" was just an exaggeration about what gets the best ratings on television and radio, but sadly, it's one-hundred percent accurate. If you want to reduce your stress levels, the worst thing you can do is tune in to something that's guaranteed to raise your blood pressure and be an unhealthy distraction, especially when it comes to politics. I've often said, "If you're more worried about who's running The White House instead of who's running your own house, then you're not going to be as positive and productive as you could be that day."

**MARCELLO'S MESSAGE:**
*"IF YOU'RE MORE WORRIED ABOUT WHO'S RUNNING THE WHITE HOUSE INSTEAD OF WHO'S RUNNING YOUR OWN HOUSE, THEN YOU'RE NOT GOING TO BE AS POSITIVE AND PRODUCTIVE AS YOU CAN BE THAT DAY."*

If you need some suggestions for a movie that will provide you with a healthy distraction, some therapeutic stress reduction, or some much-needed inspiration, here are a few of my personal favorites: *Sea Biscuit, The Blind Side, American Underdog, Rudy, GI Jane, Cinderella, Rocky I-IV, Raiders of the Lost Ark, Star Wars, Back to the Future, Dead Poets Society, Wizard of Oz, 300, Cast Away, Animal House, The Princess Bride, The Outsiders, A Night at the Museum, Forrest Gump, Ace Ventura, Field of Dreams, Karate Kid, Elf, Young Frankenstein, Anchorman, Airplane,* and of course, *Shawshank Redemption.* (*As I alluded to in* Celebrate Life, *when I finally broke through my darkest days, I felt just like Andy Duphrene at the end of* Shawshank Redemption *when he crawled face-down in a mile-long sewage pipe to break out of prison and raised his hands up in victory as the rain poured down on his body like a reinvigorating baptism.*)

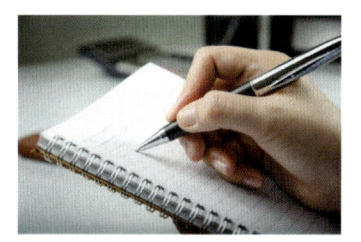

- Do you have a movie that comes to mind (newer or classic) that would be a good selection based on what you've read in the section above?

_____

_____

_____

- **SHUT UP AND LEAVE:** If you are uncomfortable at your job, at a public or private social event, or at a business meeting, to the point where your stress levels are near the boiling point— leave! Sometimes you will be surrounded by people who do not know how to disagree without being disagreeable, by people who lack the ability to agree on a sensible idea if it comes from outside of their tribe, and by people who are so entrenched in their beliefs that they are incapable of changing their opinion despite being proven wrong by science, evidence, or newly discovered facts. If this happens to you, get the heck outta there! Don't waste any more of your energy by trying to make self-righteous speeches or trying to come up with witty verbal judo comments for your social media feed. Nope, don't pass go, don't collect $200; go directly to a neutral place and chill before you say or do something stupid that will come back to haunt you thirty-seven years from now when you run for some type of office. Respectfully remove yourself from the negative and hostile situation. If you must open your mouth, try a simple, "I'm leaving now; have a nice day," or "Thank you for your time; I have nothing else to say." Your personal and professional encounters in life won't always end on a positive note with a big kumbaya hug, but you can at least learn to appreciate the stress reduction tactic and the win that comes from being able to bow out of any situation as gracefully as possible.

By the way, I always make an effort to see things from the other person's perspective regardless of how difficult or unreasonable he or she is being. Knowing I did all that I could to reach a resolution before bowing out helps me move forward with a clear conscience. Something I learned a long time ago that always gives me just enough pause when I think I'm right from the get-go and refuse to hear the other person out is the concept in this illustration shown here.

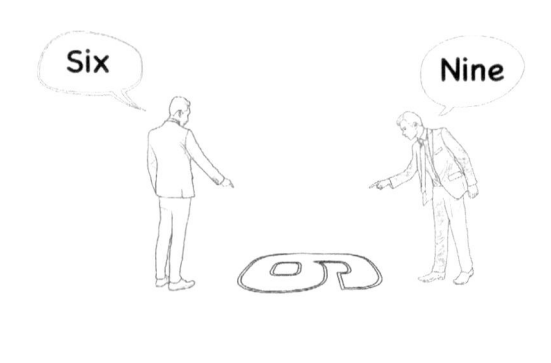

I saw a similar drawing during the early stages of the COVID-19 pandemic, when people were intensely debating whether or not to get the vaccine, to shut down schools, to close businesses, and to wear masks. I thought it was brilliant and it definitely made me reevaluate some of my opinions. The thought that two people who don't agree could both actually be right depending on their vantage point blew my mind. The magic happens in layers. In other words, during an argument, you may present facts that are based on science and research that, at their core, are fundamentally correct. However, due to extenuating circumstances and real-time updates, your stance may easily be disproven or refuted. More recently, I was listening to a great podcast by one of my favorite doctors, Peter Attia. He shared the phrase, "Strong convictions, loosely held." It's the idea that it's okay to be passionate about your beliefs and opinions and it's okay to base your stance on logic, data, and common sense. However, you can't hold on to your convictions so tightly that you become incapable of changing your mind if/when new evidence emerges that completely changes the ballgame. So, stand your ground when your heart, gut, and brain tell you do so, but like 38 Special sang in the '80s, "Hold on loosely."

The legendary motivational speaker, Dr. Wayne Dyer, once shared a very poignant parable that is meant to challenge our convictions. I thought it was a brilliant exercise in broadening our perceived boundaries. I included this not to comment on religion or the afterlife, but rather to illustrate how easy it is to become trapped by our self-imposed thought restrictions.

### LIFE AFTER DELIVERY:

*In a mother's womb were two babies. One asked the other, "Do you believe in life after delivery?"*

*The other replied, "Why, of course. There has to be something after delivery. Maybe we are here to prepare ourselves for what will be later."*

*"Nonsense," said the first. "There is no life after delivery. What kind of life would that be?"*

*The second said, "I don't know, but there will be more light than here. Maybe we will walk with our legs and eat from our mouths. Maybe we will have other senses that we can't understand now."*

*The first replied, "That is absurd. Walking is impossible. And eating with our mouths? Ridiculous! The umbilical cord supplies nutrition and everything we need. But the umbilical cord is so short. Life after delivery is to be logically excluded."*

*The second insisted, "Well I think there is something and maybe it's different than it is here. Maybe we won't need this physical cord anymore."*

*The first replied, "Nonsense. And moreover, if there is life, then why has no one ever come back from there? Delivery is the end of life, and in the after-delivery, there is nothing but darkness and silence and oblivion. It takes us nowhere."*

"Well, I don't know," said the second. "But certainly we will meet Mother and she will take care of us."

The first replied, "Mother? You actually believe in Mother? That's laughable. If Mother exists then where is She now?"

The second said, "She is all around us. We are surrounded by Her. We are of Her. It is in Her that we live. Without Her, this world would not and could not exist."

Said the first, "Well, I don't see Her, so it is only logical that She doesn't exist."

To which the second replied, "Sometimes, when you're in silence and you focus and listen, you can perceive Her presence, and you can hear Her loving voice, calling down from above."

# CHAPTER III:
# LONGEVITY

**AS DR. JILL MENTIONED IN** the last chapter, positive momentum is what speeds up recovery and increases longevity. To understand longevity, you have to understand death. I know that it's a tall order *(and frankly impossible)* to truly grasp an understanding of death. If you can at least identify the kryptonite that will kill you, then you will have a fighting chance to stave it off as long as possible while simultaneously living your best life and deliberately creating an abundant experience.

Did you know that the most common causes of death among adults and senior citizens are cancer, obesity, heart disease, diabetes, Alzheimer's, and Parkinson's Disease? Did you know that the root cause of most of these illnesses is inflammation? Yes, especially inflammation of your gut microbiome which can damage your DNA. Remember what Dr. Jill said about how sensitive the gut is to stress? Well, it's no wonder the gut microbiome would be a prime target for inflammation that leads to disease.

Here is some good news: Did you know that there is a way to reduce inflammation and prevent or delay the onset of most of these illnesses? It's called time-restricted feeding or TRF for short. *(You may have also heard it called intermittent fasting.)* In my first book, I wrote that WHAT you eat is important and HOW MUCH you eat is important, but there is a third and vital component; it's WHEN you eat. As always, timing is everything.

Before I break down what TRF is, let me first dispel two common myths.

## MYTH #1- HABIT VS. HUNGER

I've heard people say, "I have to eat three times a day. There's no way I can go a whole day without eating any food!" That's BS. Most people are eating out of habit versus hunger. I know so many people who use the drive-thru at Dunkin' or

Starbucks for coffee and a bagel every morning, not because they're starving or because they feel like they can conquer the world afterward, but simply because that's just their chosen morning routine.

Have you ever found yourself halfway through lunch or dinner and thought to yourself, "Why am I eating? I'm not even hungry," but then you proceed to finish your entire plate anyway? I have. Then you feel like total crap because it was completely avoidable and the only person to blame is yourself. Just because it's your "usual" mealtime doesn't mean you must eat. When it comes to eating, listen to your body. Don't let your mind or watch/phone dictate your hunger.

> **MARCELLO'S MESSAGE:**
> *WHEN IT COMES TO EATING, LISTEN TO YOUR BODY. DON'T LET YOUR MIND OR WATCH/PHONE DICTATE YOUR HUNGER.*

Want proof that you won't die if you skip a meal? Cool. Put both hands up above your head. Now put your hands down on either side of your belly button and squeeze. You feel that? We all have it. That's enough fat to feed you for at least two weeks. So have no fear, you will not starve to death if you skip a meal. Generally speaking, sometimes being a human with a higher-order brain is a gift and a curse. Human beings are notorious for allowing irrational anxieties to permeate their inner peace. Armed with the right knowledge, you can prevent this from happening to you.

> **MARCELLO'S MESSAGE:**
> *HUMAN BEINGS ARE NOTORIOUS FOR ALLOWING IRRATIONAL ANXIETIES TO PERMEATE THEIR INNER PEACE. ARMED WITH THE RIGHT KNOWLEDGE YOU CAN PREVENT THIS FROM HAPPENING TO YOU.*

## MYTH #2 - HUNGER VS. THIRST

I hear this a lot—"I always feel hungry." It's probably not hunger, since most of the time, it's actually thirst. Most people become so focused on food intake and calorie consumption that they ignore the vital importance of hydration. Here is a fun fact: seventy percent of people are chronically dehydrated.

### DR. JILL WILL SEE YOU NOW

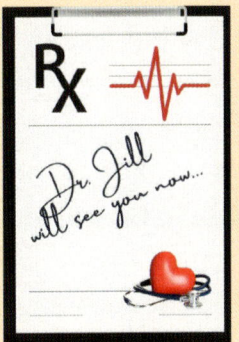

*Our early ancestors did not have readily accessible water at all times like we do, so they learned to find foods laden with water to quench their thirst, especially as they developed the evolutionary advantage of sweating. As we became modernized humans, this primitive survival mechanism of seeking out water through food sources may be playing a role in our confusion of hunger and thirst.*

*Simply refilling your water bottle a few more times, however, is not enough. Research continues to show that electrolyte deficiencies, specifically sodium (salt), potassium, and magnesium, are significant factors in developing anxiety and depression.*

*According to the FDA, most Americans consume the vast majority of dietary salt through packaged foods. However, eliminating processed foods from your diet will lower sodium intake. As we are fortunately starting to realize that processed and packaged foods are so detrimental to good health, we are also depriving ourselves of enough sodium in our diet.*

*On the other hand, getting enough potassium and magnesium is more about eating fruits, nuts, vegetables, and even animal proteins like chicken, beef, or fish. Anything green and leafy (like spinach) is generally a good source of both minerals, but you need to consume a TON of greens to hit your numbers.*

*A simple way to fix these challenges is to add electrolytes to your water, especially when exercising. These days there are several high-quality, sugar-free flavored electrolyte supplement powders that go right in your water which can help you replenish your stores and make plain old water taste a little better. I'm a big fan of a company called LMNT.*

So here's what you need to know about time-restricted feeding. TRF allows your gastrointestinal system, liver, and pancreas to take a break from digesting food. Most people are snacking and eating constantly throughout the day, and the body never has a chance to catch up. Not eating for extended periods allows insulin levels to go down low enough and long enough so you can start to burn your stored fat for energy.

This is where ketosis comes in. Burning ketones is a more efficient way of burning fuel. Dr. Jill and I are big fans of combining the ketogenic-based nutrition plan with time-restricted feeding. If you want a super-detailed explanation and deep dive into all this, you can invest a few hours and read *The Obesity Code* by Dr. Jason Fung and *Bulletproof* by Dave Asprey. The short version is that TRF allows your body to turn off digestion and focus on clearing toxins and damaged cells. A magical thing called autophagy happens when your body has a chance to clean house. Autophagy literally means to "eat thyself." Autophagy protects your brain and enhances brain function by eating up those damaged cells that would otherwise build up and lead to neurodegenerative diseases like Alzheimer's and dementia. Autophagy also helps lower the risk of cancer, heart disease, arthritis, and asthma. The moral of the story? Autophagy is good for you. Go get some!

Before you do, know this—everybody's body is different. Be sure to pay close attention and listen to yours.

**MARCELLO'S MESSAGE:**
*EVERYBODY'S BODY IS DIFFERENT. BE SURE TO PAY CLOSE ATTENTION AND LISTEN TO YOURS.*

First, consult with your doctor and get some blood work done, and, if possible, have your stool analyzed so you can see what's happening inside your body. If you are diabetic, have a history of disordered eating, or if you are a woman, particularly during pregnancy and your monthly cycle, you will definitely require a more specialized approach to time-restricted feeding. That said, if you're a candidate, here are some popular options:

## THE 16/8

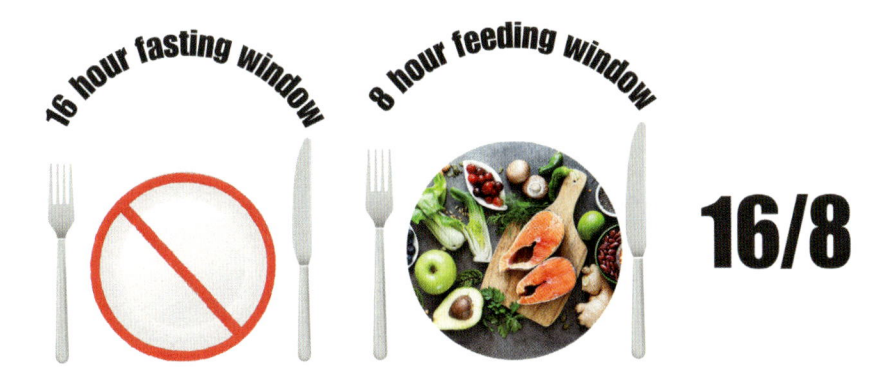

This is the most common form of TRF for beginners. All you need to do is skip breakfast or dinner. The goal is to fast for sixteen hours and have an eight-hour window for eating. Most people I know and most of my lifestyle clients simply skip breakfast, then eat lunch around 11:00 am and then have dinner around 7:00 p.m. This is a great option if you have kids or people with whom you enjoy eating dinner. If you really love starting your day with breakfast, however, no worries. You can still reap the benefits of the 16/8 by enjoying breakfast around 9:00 a.m. and then having a later lunch around 4:00 p.m. Eating "only" two meals per day and not snacking before, in between, or afterward might seem extreme when you think of the normal daily food intake for an American. However, when you realize just how many excess calories you've been eating and just how unhealthy some of your old habits were, your eyes will be opened to a whole new world of self-care.

**MARCELLO'S MESSAGE:**
*WHEN YOU REALIZE JUST HOW MANY EXCESS CALORIES YOU'VE BEEN EATING AND JUST HOW UNHEALTHY SOME OF YOUR OLD HABITS WERE, YOUR EYES WILL BE OPENED TO A WHOLE NEW WORLD OF SELF-CARE.*

## THE O.M.A.D.

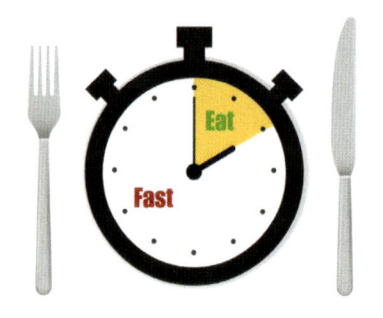

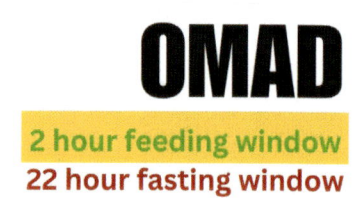

**OMAD**
2 hour feeding window
22 hour fasting window

This is an advanced form of time-restricted feeding. O.M.A.D. stands for One Meal a Day. Would you like to have breakfast, lunch, or dinner? Pick one because that's the meal where all of your calories for the day will be consumed. Now, before you start thinking that one meal is never going to be enough to satisfy your hunger, please know that, when executed correctly, your portions for this one meal are going to be noticeably larger and enough to support a well-rounded intake of healthy calories.

The O.M.A.D. definitely takes more discipline than the 16/8 and might take a couple of weeks or months to work up to. Over the years, my body seems to respond best to making my one meal for the day a late lunch around 3:00 p.m. You will need to experiment with which meal will work for your personal preferences.

One of the awesome benefits about having multiple options is that you can always mix things up from week to week or month to month to keep it interesting and to keep your body metabolically flexible. The reality is, as most of you know, life happens. You're going to need to be able to adapt without falling apart. There will be family events, outings with friends, or lunch meetings that might throw off your TRF plan on a particular day. Don't sweat it.

If you've got children, well, you know how unpredictable things can get with their after-school schedule or getting sick from some other kids in their class who don't know how to cover their noses when they sneeze. Just do your best to stay on track as consistently as possible and try not to beat yourself up when your six-day streak of being on point with everything gets interrupted. You may be tempted to say to yourself, "Well, my little wellness/self-care routine got mangled today unexpectedly, so I might as well take a death spiral into the depths of gluttony for the next nine days!" (*Not that I've ever personally said that or wanted to do that or actually tried that and totally enjoyed the first three days!*) However, the most important thing you can do is forgive yourself for being imperfect (*because, hey, newsflash, we are all imperfect*), pick yourself up from where you left off, and start your next day by saying to yourself, "Onwards and upwards!" By the way, the same philosophy applies if/when your workout routine gets thrown off.

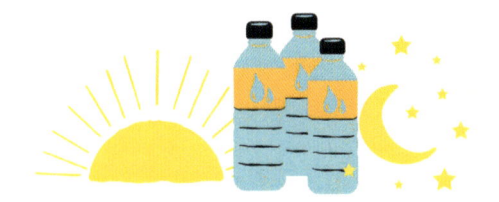

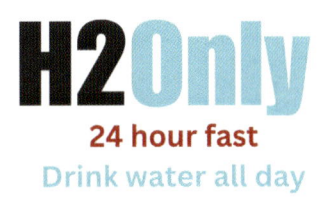

## THE H2ONLY

The H2Only is an expert form of TRF. It means what it says; the only thing you will be eating or drinking for the entire day will be water. Don't worry, you only do this for a set time frame at various times of the year. This could be from one to three days up to five to seven days.

The five-to-seven-day option will result in maximum autophagy. I recommend that you look into this and do it at least once or twice per year as a wellness reset. Dr. Jill and I usually do a five-day or seven-day H2Only fast in November right before Thanksgiving and another in the spring around Easter. You better like drinking water or learn to like drinking water because you'll need to drink about three liters each day when you're not eating. You also better make sure that if you aren't used to drinking about three liters of water each day, you stay close to a bathroom throughout the day because you'll be peeing more often. If you are like me, a guy who normally has to pee twenty-seven times per day, keeping a pee cup/container in your car will be mandatory.

Anywho, here are three reasons why you should consider doing an H2Only if you're a candidate:

- **YOU'LL GET TO SEE JUST HOW MENTALLY TOUGH YOU ARE.** Look, skipping a meal for a few hours or a whole day really isn't that big of a deal. However, not eating for multiple days can be a real mind-bender. Unless you give up at hour eighteen or on day two at lunchtime, you'll be amazed at just how much untapped mental toughness reserves you have within you. This realization at the end of a scheduled fast is priceless.

> **MARCELLO'S MESSAGE:**
> YOU'LL BE AMAZED AT JUST HOW MUCH UNTAPPED MENTAL TOUGHNESS RESERVES YOU HAVE WITHIN YOU. THIS REALIZATION AT THE END OF A SCHEDULED FAST IS PRICELESS.

- **YOU'LL APPRECIATE YOUR MEALS AGAIN.** When you finish a multiple-day fast, your first meal will be glorious. Your taste buds will have reset, and you will enjoy every morsel of what you eat. Even something as simple as beef bone broth (*one of the recommended meals to safely end a fast and re-introduce food to your system*) will taste amazing. Go one step further in your meal appreciation enhancement and practice putting your fork or spoon down between bites. This habit will serve you well for the rest of your life.

- **YOU WILL REALIZE THAT EATING THREE TIMES PER DAY WITH SNACKS IN BETWEEN IS UNNECESSARY.** The only reason you eat so much is because that's what modern society, food manufacturers, or family members told you was the norm. Once you figure this out and allow yourself to break this obesity-inducing habit, you will unlock a powerful new door to a more intelligent self-care routine.

Time-restricted feeding is a win-win. Many of you might be aware that a positive side effect of TRF is weight loss. While dropping a few pounds of fat and fitting into your favorite jeans again feels really good, that's not even the best part. Nope. Not even close. For starters, TRF will save you money and time. You'll spend less money on groceries and less time shopping, whether it's online or at the supermarket. In addition, you'll spend less time sitting down to eat three or four meals per day and less time waiting at the drive-thru for some greasy food that will probably upset your stomach anyway.

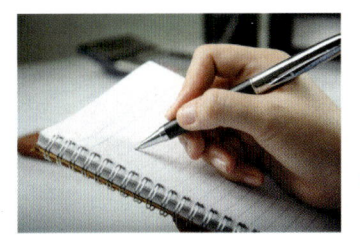

Now that you've learned time-restricted feeding can save you time and money:

- What would you do with the extra time?

_____
_____
_____

- What would you do with the extra money?

_____
_____
_____

Like the old Ginsu Knife commercials always said, "But wait, there's more!" In my opinion, one of the greatest benefits of time-restricted feeding is that you will actually have more energy. In the next chapter, I will discuss why Ralph Waldo Emerson was right when he said, "The world belongs to the energetic."

## CHAPTER IV:
# ENERGY

**REMEMBER IN THE LAST CHAPTER** how I discussed how time-restricted feeding can help increase ketone production in the body? Well, when you burn ketones for energy, it's a more efficient process than the body's default mechanism of burning carbohydrates for energy. The net result is more energy. When you have more energy, it is easier to do more weight training. The more weight training you do, the more muscle you will build. The more muscle you build, the easier it is to maintain and increase your balance, stability, and flexibility.

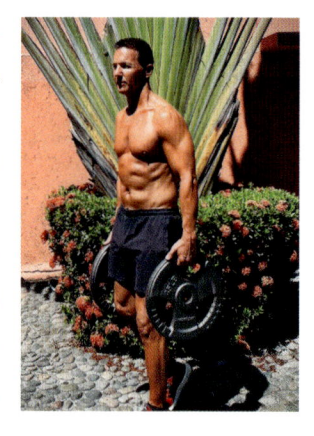

> **MARCELLO'S MESSAGE:**
> THE MORE MUSCLE YOU BUILD, THE EASIER IT IS TO MAINTAIN AND INCREASE YOUR BALANCE, STABILITY, AND FLEXIBILITY.

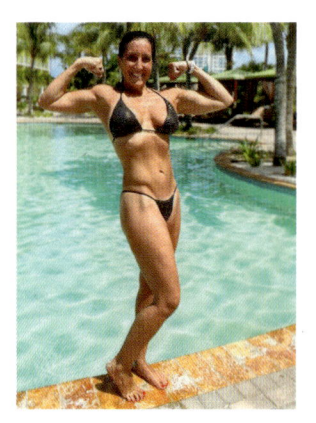

Some of you who follow me on social media might know that Dr. Jill and I work out a lot, but it *really* is for more than the reasons you may think. Spoiler alert: Working out gives us the energy we need to train for the Olympics. No, not for the upcoming Summer or Winter Olympics, but for the Senior Olympics twenty-five years from now. And the gold medal for winning? Longevity and high quality of life!

## DR. JILL WILL SEE YOU NOW

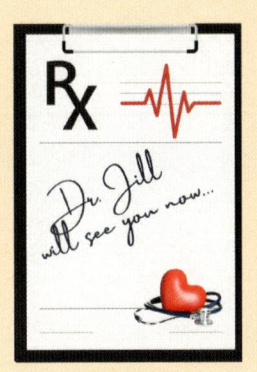

There is a very real thing that happens to all of us as we age called sarcopenia, basically muscle breakdown or muscle wasting. This can definitely put a damper on your Olympic success. Unfortunately, it starts when we are young, around thirty years old, and we continue to naturally lose muscle mass (and strength) each year going forward. Making sure to increase dietary protein and having a consistent weight training routine as we age are critical to preserving as much muscle mass as we can. No matter what path your life takes you down, please make a conscious effort to invest in your physical health as much as you do your business, family, and hobbies.

Now that you know one of the main medical reasons why you should train (*to prevent or delay sarcopenia*), let me give you some practical and real-life reasons why you want to start training now for your Senior Olympics. (**This longevity concept was brought to my attention by Dr. Peter Attia, whom I mentioned earlier and who knows a lot about the subject.**)

Just like a decathlon, you'll be competing in ten events:

- Going up a flight of stairs with a fifteen-pound bag of groceries in each hand
- Getting up and down out of a chair
- Getting in and out of a car
- Getting up off the floor after playing with your grandkids
- Getting yourself back up unassisted after an unexpected fall
- Cooking basic meals
- Walking to the end of the driveway to put out the trash
- Dusting and vacuuming your home
- Transferring your own laundry from the washer to the dryer
- Showering on your own

These are just a few basic physical activities that you will need in order to navigate daily life safely and independently as a senior citizen. They are also activities that almost all of us take for granted when we have youth on our side. Maintaining proportionate and sufficient levels of strength, balance, and flexibility as you age will help you preserve your independence and quality of life as long as possible.

> **MARCELLO'S MESSAGE:**
> *MAINTAINING PROPORTIONATE AND SUFFICIENT LEVELS OF STRENGTH, BALANCE, AND FLEXIBILITY AS YOU AGE WILL HELP YOU PRESERVE YOUR INDEPENDENCE AND QUALITY OF LIFE AS LONG AS POSSIBLE.*

Whether or not you get featured on the cover of a Wheaties cereal box for your performance in your Senior Olympics, there are a few other honorable mention categories in which you'll want to do well. Some of the happiest seniors I know are still actively social, show plenty of affection to friends and loved ones, and are enthusiastic about traveling abroad or even just outside their comfort zone.

Folks like Norma and Ken Kahn, our dear friends and neighbors in Costa Rica, embody the spirit of Senior Olympian gold medalists. They hike the mountain each morning, swim every afternoon, walk their groceries up four flights of stairs, belong to the local book club, entertain friends on Fridays for Shabbat dinner, and still travel to different countries. (*They were very excited to tell us about their upcoming trip to Morocco that they have scheduled on their calendar!*) When they travel, they must compete in one of the Senior Olympic events in which Dr. Jill and I want to excel—being able to lift a twenty-five-pound carry-on suitcase and put it in the overhead compartment of the plane without causing a huge line of passengers behind them.

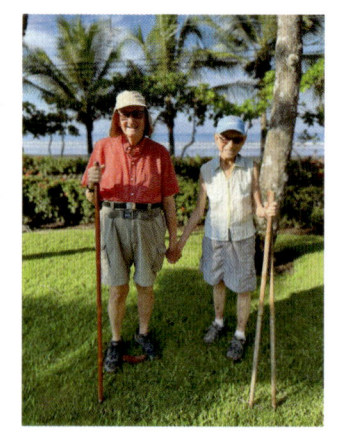

Speaking of traveling, how about getting your passport at ninety years old like my father-in-law, Frank Garripoli? Despite having arthritis and outliving his wife of sixty-three years, Frank still joins us each year in Costa Rica for a week

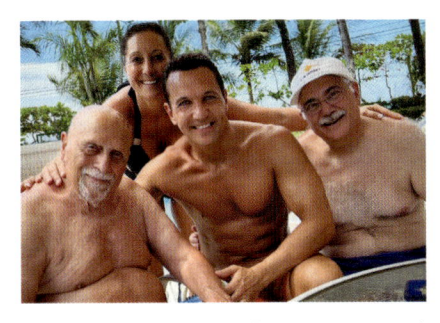

*(with Frank, Jill, and my Dad in Costa Rica, 2023)*

to swim, sail, and play three fierce games of Yahtzee each night. Frank also rides in the support van with my dad for our annual Celebrate Life bike rides in New York and New Jersey. Speaking of my dad, a true Senior Olympic champion like Vic Pedalino does all of the above; plus he volunteers a few times each week for great causes like Habitat for Humanity and his local food bank.

Whether you are training for the Olympics or not, I want you to wake up in the morning feeling like an Olympic champion. It all boils down to purpose and passion, two tenets of fulfillment confirmed by Dan Buettner's extensive research in *The Blue Zones of Happiness*. I want you to have enough energy and fire in your belly to wake up having:

> Something to do
> Someone to love
> Something to give
> Something to look forward to
> Something to believe in

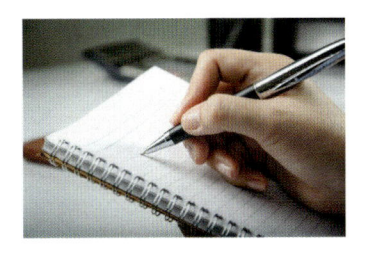

**MARCELLO'S MESSAGE:**
*WAKE UP HAVING SOMETHING TO DO, SOMEONE TO LOVE, SOMETHING TO GIVE, SOMETHING TO LOOK FORWARD TO, AND SOMETHING TO BELIEVE IN.*

Let's find out more about your purpose in life and the source of your passion.

- What is something that motivates you to get up and out of bed each morning?

  _____
  _____

- Who is someone you can express your love to every day?

  _____
  _____

- What is something you can give your time and energy to every day?

  _____
  _____

- What is something you can look forward to doing today or in the near future?

  _____
  _____

- What is something you believe in?

  _____
  _____

Turn the page to Chapter five to see how you can increase your odds of waking up feeling like an Olympic champion.

## CHAPTER V:
# SLEEP

**HIGH-QUALITY SLEEP IS VITAL TO** your chances of waking up feeling like an Olympic champion. It is important to be as consistent as you possibly can. Like stress reduction, proper sleep is crucial for living your best life. From this moment forward, how can you get better sleep?

The first thing I recommend is to develop the best sleep hygiene possible. This starts in the morning by getting adequate exposure to sunlight whenever it is available to help set your circadian rhythm. Later in the day, stop eating at least three hours before bedtime so that your body has time to digest. Sleep can then be dedicated to cellular housekeeping and immune system repair. In addition, limiting screens before bed is important.

Here are five of my personal sleep hygiene tips to ensure the best quality sleep each night:

- **ELIMINATE THE BLUE LIGHT:** If you weren't already aware, the blue light emitted from screens is the same wavelength as the midday sun, and it constantly tricks our brains into thinking it is daytime. Make sure you put down the phone and shut off the TV at least one hour prior to bedtime. Even better, get rid of the TV in your bedroom to eliminate the temptation of turning it on when you are trying to fall asleep or in the middle of the night when you can't sleep.

- **INSTALL BLACKOUT CURTAINS:** Instead of regular curtains, hang blackout curtains over your windows. This is a great way to create a dark and quiet sleep space.

- **SET BOUNDARIES:** Allowing your children to sleep in your bed and/or bedroom is a great way to prevent yourself from getting a good night's rest and decrease the opportunity to be intimate with your partner.

## DR. JILL WILL SEE YOU NOW

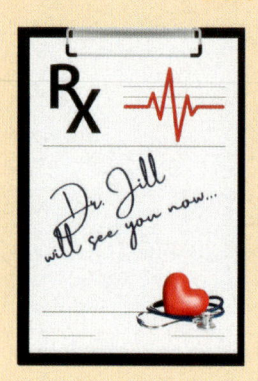

We cannot ignore two facts about our early ancestors: family groups all huddled up in the same cave at night for protection against predators in the dark, and infants stayed with their mothers for at least the full first year of life. In addition, crying was the only tool infants had (and have today) to ensure their needs were met. Humans are hardwired to respond to an infant crying, which is a great evolutionary method to ensure survival of the species. The concept of families staying together at night for survival has been passed down in our collective consciousness as humans throughout history. In addition to the modern demand of both parents working during the day, it is no wonder why so many parents have a difficult time handling a crying infant at night—they are fighting against millions of years of human evolution.

If there is one aspect of life where we **should** be selfish, it is the need to prioritize a good night's sleep. That is why it is so important to help our babies learn to sleep early and effectively—so we can sleep, too! Parents, especially moms, are putting their own needs on the back burner. They are allowing their desire to be a good parent by "protecting" their baby from crying to overshadow their need to take care of themselves.

A relatively recent study published in the journal, **Pediatrics**, found that sleep training DOES NOT cause long-term harm to babies. The study refutes a 2012 study wherein the authors concluded that allowing a baby to cry for extended periods raised stress levels. No parent wants to cause their child discomfort or, worse, raise their stress levels, but chronic sleep deprivation suffered by both parents and their poor sleeper inevitably affects the family's entire life. That, I promise, raises everyone's stress levels.

As a proper sleep routine starts to take shape, the paradigm will inevitably shift from feeling selfish (I need my sleep) to selfless (I gave my child an incredibly valuable lifetime tool— the ability to self-soothe), and then the ripple effect begins. Better sleep leads to happier family members, more productivity at work, more energy to be the best parent possible, and an overall improvement in the parents' physical and mental well-being. I would never pretend that there is a quick fix to sleep training since every baby is different, every parent is unique, and every family dynamic is blissfully complex in its own way. However, once parents face the reality of their situation and tease out the excuses from the fears, they find the strength to take back the night and help their child learn to figure it out and get some rest.

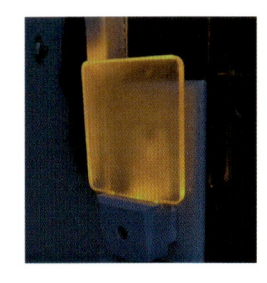

- **USE AN AMBER GLOW NIGHT LIGHT:** Most of us will get up at night to use the bathroom, and just a few minutes of exposure to the light emitted from a traditional night light can cause a disruption in our sleep for the rest of the night. The glow of an amber-colored night light instead of a regular night light will keep you sleepy by helping you feel calm and promote the body's natural secretion of melatonin. They sell them on Amazon for just a few bucks.

- **USE A SLEEP CROWN PILLOW:** One of the most helpful sleep hacks Dr. Jill and I have come across is a sleep crown pillow. It acts like an oversized sleep mask filled with feathers that buffer out sound and light to help you sleep like a rock.

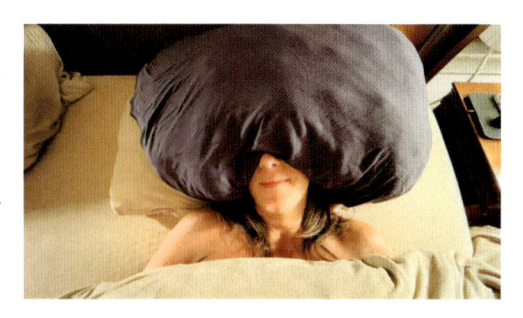

In addition to ensuring the highest quality sleep, ideally, you want to track your sleep and get feedback because, as some people we admire often say, what gets measured gets managed. Even further, what gets measured frequently improves quickly.

### MARCELLO'S MESSAGE:

*WHAT GETS MEASURED GETS MANAGED. WHAT GETS MEASURED FREQUENTLY IMPROVES QUICKLY.*

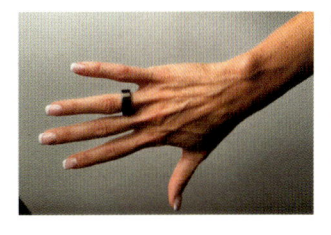

Since we are unconscious when we sleep, it is oftentimes difficult to tell if we got a good night's sleep or not. Your recollection of your sleep quality may not reflect what actually happened. There are a lot of apps and devices on the market to track sleep. For years, my wife has been wearing an Oura ring.

> ### DR. JILL WILL SEE YOU NOW
>
> An Oura ring is a fabulous tool that not only gives me real-time data on my daily step count and movement/recovery balance, but it helps me track my deep and REM sleep. While humans spend most of the night in light sleep, we need to have a good balance of deep and REM sleep cycles throughout the night as well. We get most of our deep sleep (the most restorative and rejuvenating phase of sleep when muscles grow and repair and the immune system refreshes) in the first half of the night, and REM sleep (the phase associated with dreaming, memory consolidation, and creativity) in the second half of the night. The percent of our night spent in each phase naturally decreases as we age, so it is vitally important to use all of the tools available to "stack the deck," as our friend Randy Bartlett says, and preserve as much deep and REM sleep as we can.
>
> Many people will say that they get their "eight hours" because their schedule allows them to either go to sleep very early and wake up at 3:00 a.m. or stay up until 3:00 a.m. and not wake up until later in the morning. I mentioned above that deep and REM sleep each happen at specific times of the night. News flash—going to sleep later but waking up later (or vice versa)—will eventually throw off the deep/REM balance and can build irreversible sleep debt. It's more about quality than quantity.

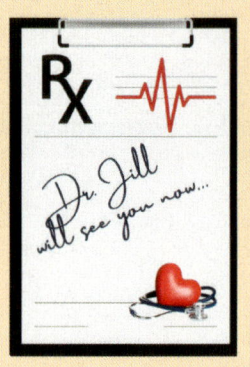

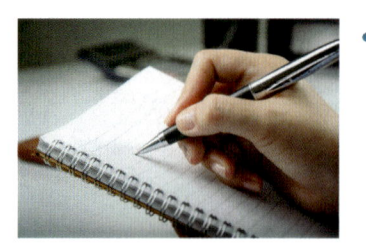

- Based on the information above, what are three things you can do to improve your daily sleep quality and overall sleep hygiene?

_____
_____
_____

## CHAPTER VI:
# PHYSICAL ENVIRONMENT

**IN THE PREVIOUS FIVE CHAPTERS,** I laid out a solid foundation for moving onwards and upwards and living your best life from today forward. The building blocks of this foundation are:

- **Stress Reduction**
- **Nutrition**
- **Exercise**
- **Sleep**

Now, let's focus on creating the optimal environment so you can effectively support and maintain your lifestyle evolution— because if you can change your environment, you can change your life.

> **MARCELLO'S MESSAGE:**
> *CHANGE YOUR ENVIRONMENT, CHANGE YOUR LIFE.*

Do you really feel that you have optimized your personal environment to make you the fittest, healthiest, and most productive person you can be? If so, good for you! Whether we like it or not (*or know it or not*), we all have to come to terms with the fact that we alone are responsible for creating the life we are living. Most people do it passively and unconsciously, but Dr. Jill and I want to be deliberate creators and I want you to be one, too. In her first children's book, *The Universe*

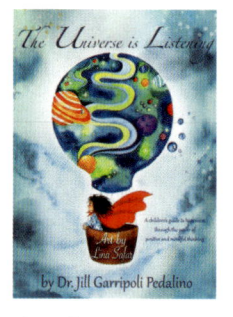

*Is Listening: A Children's Guide to Happiness Through the Power of Positive and Mindful Thinking*, that was the message for the kids. Turns out, parents and other adults said they needed to hear that message just as much as the kids did. Deliberate creation includes consciously sculpting our physical environment, interpersonal environment, financial environment, and, perhaps most importantly, our emotional environment.

The first component of the environment that we're going to focus on is physical (*your living space and your workspace*).

For your home office or business location, I highly recommend a stand-up desk. One of my favorite expressions coined by author Nilofer Merchant, "Sitting is the new smoking," is not only catchy, but it's fairly accurate. Let's take it one step further and say, even more accurately, that *inactivity* is the new smoking. Sitting is not necessarily bad, but between driving, working at a desk, and watching TV, most Americans spend just about the entire day sitting or physically stagnant. I like the positive spin that my friend, Neen, put on it when she suggested, "Standing is the new standard."

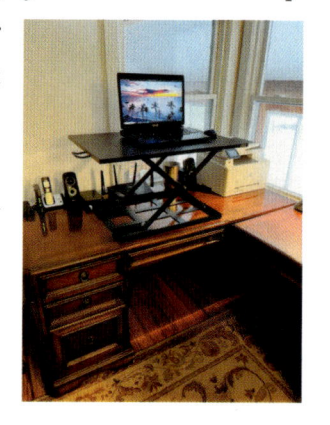

If you want to reduce back pain, improve circulation, and stay focused longer, a stand-up desk is a great investment. Don't worry about not having enough energy to stand all day if you've always been a sitter, or are not in the best shape right now. Like a new weight training or cardio program, you can start slowly and incrementally build up your stamina or simply do a hybrid plan where you stand for twenty minutes and then lower the desk to sit for the next forty minutes. Eventually, you'll likely find yourself flipping the ratio by standing for forty and sitting for twenty. There's a reason why some of the most successful people have meetings standing up or even while walking. A stand-up desk keeps you on your toes and prevents that awful lethargic feeling that results from being immobile for too long.

> **MARCELLO'S MESSAGE:**
> *SITTING IS THE NEW SMOKING. STANDING IS THE NEW STANDARD.*

For your kitchen, make it a point to surround yourself with the right fuel. Do the tough job of taking inventory of your fridge and kitchen cabinets (*or hire a professional to help*) and eliminate the processed and sugary foods that fill the cupboards of most American kitchens. These products, intentionally made to be addictive and tempting by huge food manufacturing companies, are responsible for much of the current obesity epidemic in our country.

We talked about the importance of building muscle to prevent sarcopenia. If you want to build muscle, you'll need an appropriate amount of quality protein in your nutrition plan. ButcherBox is one of our favorite sources of grass-fed and grass-finished animal protein that can be delivered monthly to your doorstep. By the way, we've done the math, and ButcherBox ends up costing about the same as high-quality store-bought lean protein. Remember, you are what you eat—when you consume the meat of a stressed-out, steroid-filled cow, chicken, or pig from an industrial feedlot, you are ingesting all those stress hormones and harmful chemicals. It may not always be possible, convenient, or financially practical to buy the highest quality protein, but just make an effort when you can to consistently seek out the best sources of protein. Simply being more aware of what you put into your mouth is a meaningful first step.

> **MARCELLO'S MESSAGE:**
> *YOU ARE WHAT YOU EAT. WHEN YOU CONSUME STRESSED-OUT ANIMALS, YOU CONSUME THEIR STRESS.*

Too busy to cook or buy your groceries? No worries. Check out companies like Eat Clean Bro that deliver beautiful, precooked meals to your home each week. If you can do your math and find that meal delivery options are financially comparable to the gas, time, and expense of buying food at the store, go for it. Do whatever works best for your situation.

For your dinner table, try these two house rules that have become staples for our family at home:

### RULE #1

No phones at the dinner table. Period. You need to set an example for your kids. Look, if you can't sit at the table without checking your phone for an entire meal, you need help because you are probably addicted—and that's no joke.

### RULE # 2

No complaining. Well, it's more like you're not allowed to complain for more than three minutes if you don't have a solution or you're not interested in a solution. Although mealtime is a great time to catch up with your kids and loved ones about what's happening, don't allow excessive complaining to disrupt that precious quality time. Of course, it's okay to vent and share your frustration about a challenge you are experiencing, but at a certain point, you begin to spend more energy on the problem than on the solution. In any home (*or anywhere for that matter*), remember this one principle: complaining kills momentum; solutions create momentum.

**MARCELLO'S MESSAGE:**
*COMPLAINING KILLS MOMENTUM; SOLUTIONS CREATE MOMENTUM.*

## CHAPTER VII:
# INTERPERSONAL ENVIRONMENT

**HUMANS ARE SOCIAL CREATURES DESIGNED** to engage in relationships with one another. While they can be uplifting and enriching, certain relationships can also be an anchor that weighs you down and prevents you from living your best life. Before you go to work changing up your social circle, take a good look in the mirror. As a pediatrician, Dr. Jill has her own unique perspective on this topic.

### DR. JILL WILL SEE YOU NOW

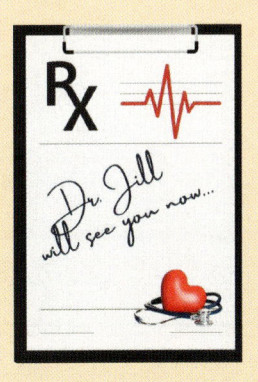

*When it comes to the interpersonal component, I'll ask you a question I ask all my patients at their yearly checkups. Whether they are three years old or twenty-three years old, I will end my visit with, "Who is the most important person in your life?"*

*At my practice, in an effort to give me the "right" answer (which is why they lie to me about all the vegetables they eat), the kids offer answers like, "The most important person in my life is my grandma, my parents, God, my dog..." The real answer is—it's YOU!*

*The most important relationship in the world is between you and the inner you. You can't offer anyone anything meaningful if you're out of alignment. As my husband always says, "If you can't take care of yourself, you can't take care of the people who depend on you."*

*If you have kids and/or a partner, you have multiple other relationships to nurture so you need to figure yourself out first. By the way, speaking of*

> relationships, I hear this one a lot—happy wife, happy life (the idea that your happiness depends on your wife or spouse's happiness). I call BS. Do you want to know why? Well, I'll say it again; you can't offer anyone anything meaningful if you are out of alignment. Oh, you can stand on your head for that other person, but if you're not first thinking about what makes you happy then you will end up failing every time. This is not selfish; this is selfless. As a woman, I can tell you that "happy wife, happy life" is a BS rule. Please keep in mind that many of the rules we do follow were made by those no smarter than us. This is not to say don't follow the Golden Rule (treat others as you want to be treated and, of course, don't kill anybody), but absolutely challenge the heck out of the rest!

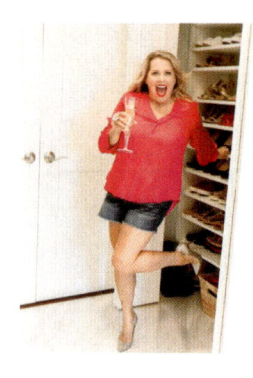

You've probably heard me say, "You need to keep good company" and "You are who you surround yourself with." In *Celebrate Life*, I talked about VIPs and VDPs, a concept introduced to me by my luxuriously stilettoed Aussie friend and mentor, Neen James. VIPs are **VERY INSPIRATIONAL PEOPLE**. They are people who will tell you what you need to hear, not just what you want to hear. Just the opposite, VDPs are **VERY DRAINING PEOPLE**. These are the toxic people who can come up with a problem to every solution.

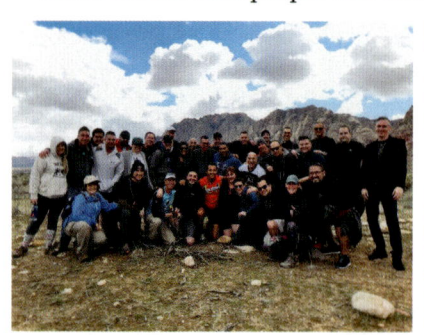

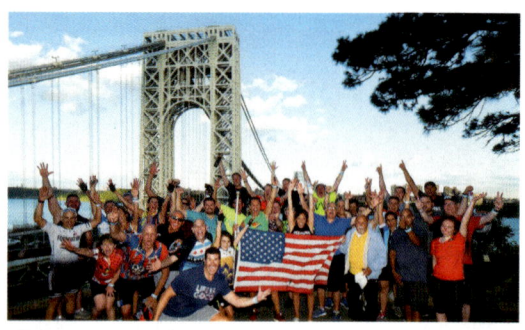

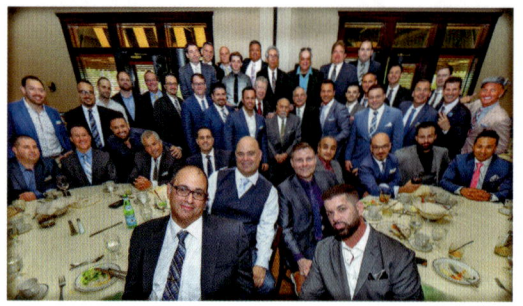

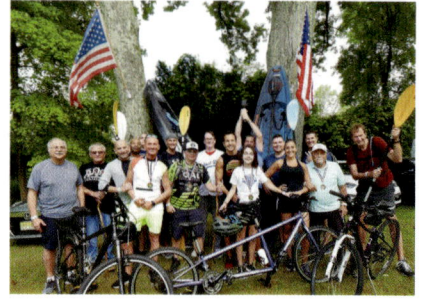

Many of you might be familiar with the annual hikes, bike rides, outdoor adventures, and lunches I organize. This is my way of deliberately creating a positive and productive environment. And you can do the same. You just need one or two solid VIPs to get the ball rolling.

How do you find your VIPs? You need to ask yourself two questions. The first question is, "With whom do I need to start spending more time?" (*Seek out individuals who you observe online or in person doing awesome things or displaying an exemplary attitude that is above and beyond the usual blasé and jaded energy running rampant in our society.*) The second question is, "With whom do I need to stop spending time?" (*I believe in addition by subtraction, so removing one very draining person from your life can be just as valuable as adding two very inspirational people.*)

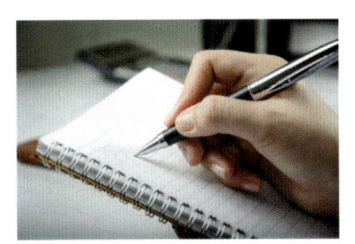

Based on what you've just read about VIPs and VDPs:

- With whom do you need to start spending more time?

_____

_____

_____

- With whom do you need to start spending less time?

_____

_____

_____

The goal is to find a veraciously honest accountability partner. In addition to telling you what you need to hear and not just what you want to hear, that person should be someone who embodies a healthy dose of the old school "tough love" philosophy mixed with just enough genuine and authentic compassion to keep you moving onwards and upwards. Veracious honesty is essential if you want to reach your full potential. Be prepared for the advice to sting from time to time.

However, you will find that in many cases, the advice was something you already knew but were just not admitting to yourself.

> **MARCELLO'S MESSAGE:**
> *VERACIOUS HONESTY IS ESSENTIAL IF YOU WANT TO REACH YOUR FULL POTENTIAL.*

When it comes to finding a spouse or significant other, look for a worthy partner, and don't settle for anything less than the soulmate you deserve. I think Cindi Sansone-Braff, the author of *Grant Me A Higher Love*, nailed it when she wrote:

> "... Soulmates see eye to eye on most important issues and they agree to disagree on others with no ill effects. They have a great many interests in common and this makes them not only lovers, but best friends as well. These couples can withstand the winds of change and they seem to be able to face every situation in life, no matter how harsh, with grace and courage. For this reason, people tend to look up to them for inspiration. Soulmates tend to have passionate relationships, not only with each other, but with the rest of the world. They are active and passionate participators in life. Often times these couples join forces to fight for a cause they believe in and this benefits not only their local community, but the larger world as well. At the end of their lives, they'll feel they have accomplished almost everything they wanted and needed to do, and they know they have each other to thank for this. As long as both soulmates are alive, no one on earth can take the place of the other."

# CHAPTER VIII:
# FINANCIAL ENVIRONMENT

**WHEN IT COMES TO CREATING** your financial environment, this takes just as much awareness as when you are creating your physical and interpersonal environments. There is a strong connection between recovery, stress reduction, and eliminating the burden of debt. In *Celebrate Life*, I mentioned one of America's most popular personal finance experts, Dave Ramsey. You may have heard him say that some people only change their financial environment by default because they are literally "sick and tired of being sick and tired" of being in debt. I, myself, am a big Dave Ramsey fan and I learned from Dave and personal experience that if you reduce your debt, you definitely reduce your stress. Like the fictional Mexican fisherman and some of our friends in Costa Rica, it is possible for you to make half as much money, but be twice as happy. You may have to live in a smaller house, drive an older car, or not buy that new outfit you saw in the store, but guess what? Some of the most truly successful people I know recognize the difference between the fleeting high that comes from buying material things versus the lasting value of memories and experiences money cannot buy.

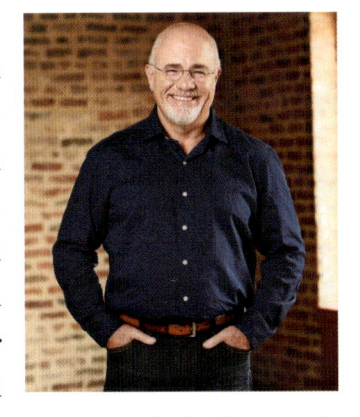

**MARCELLO'S MESSAGE:** *RECOGNIZE THE DIFFERENCE BETWEEN THE FLEETING HIGH THAT COMES FROM BUYING MATERIAL THINGS VERSUS THE LASTING VALUE OF MEMORIES AND EXPERIENCES MONEY CANNOT BUY.*

### DR. JILL WILL SEE YOU NOW

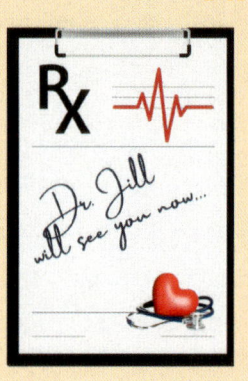

My particular path in life led me to accumulate over $200,000 in school debt. I also had a monthly car payment and mortgages on not one, but two multi-family properties that I purchased at the height of the housing market. Marcello shared with me when we first started dating some of the principles he learned from listening to Dave Ramsey's radio show. As a result, I started giving every dollar a name and kept working my butt off in my new practice. Within two years, I paid off the school loan, sold the properties, got rid of the lease, and bought a used car. When I eliminated the debt, I felt great! My savings account was empty, but the stress reduction alone was worth its weight in gold. Another positive side effect was that I was now able to help build our savings. Within a few more years, we had enough cash to jump on an opportunity to buy a beautiful Costa Rican beachfront condo, which we love to visit each year.

While we are not by any means financial advisors, here are four of the main tips that keep Dr. Jill and me, as Dave says, in "financial peace":

- **DON'T BUY SOMETHING THAT YOU CANNOT AFFORD.** If you want a crash course in financial peace and a good laugh, go on YouTube and check out the comedy sketch from Saturday Night Live called "Don't Buy Stuff You Cannot Afford." This doesn't mean you have to cut up all your credit cards and live like a monk in Tibet with no material possessions. However, if you don't have the money in the bank to pay for it outright, you will seriously want to reconsider the urgency of the purchase. An easy litmus test to know if the purchase is financially practical is to ask yourself, "Do I *need* this, or do I *want* this?" If it is not something urgent like new brakes for your car, then it is probably best to pause and revisit the potential purchase at a later date. Prioritizing necessities over desires is paramount.

- **ELIMINATE OR PAY DOWN YOUR DEBT AS SOON AS POSSIBLE.**
  It's not just about earning the desirable position of having a zero balance on your credit card. More importantly, it is about the sense of freedom and calm that comes with going to bed not having to worry about where the money is going to come for the next bill. As I mentioned, be prepared to make some sacrifices or meaningful lifestyle adjustments. There is no magic wand or genie in a bottle that will make your debt instantly disappear. Unless you are fortunate enough to have a trust fund or win the lottery, maintaining financial autonomy takes discipline and a long-term commitment.
- **SET A GOAL.** Whether you are focused on reducing your school loans or saving for a condo in Costa Rica, know why you are working towards your financial goal. Having something to focus on allows you to understand why you are working so hard or temporarily eliminating short-term satisfaction for long-term reward.
- **HIRE A PROFESSIONAL.** There are plenty of sleazy and corrupt financial professionals out there, but if you can find a solid accountant and advisor, they can have a meaningful impact on your current and future financial situation. Like many things in life, you don't know what you don't know. Although you might be able to cruise through life without the assistance of someone who knows a lot more than you do about things like retirement funds, college savings plans, health savings accounts, lesser-known tax deductions, alternative asset classes, and why it's probably best to stay away from some shady stuff like Bitcoin (*unless you want to end up on the next episode of* American Greed), please consider getting some professional help.

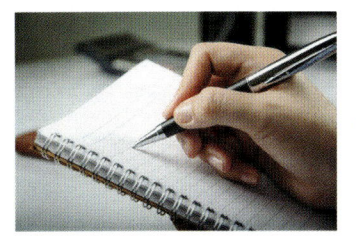

Name a reoccurring expense or source of debt you have that is a want vs. a need.

- Which aspect of personal finance are you good at?

_____

_____

- Which aspect of personal finance could you improve upon?

_____

_____

# CHAPTER IX:
# EMOTIONAL ENVIRONMENT

**THE ANCIENT CHINESE PHILOSOPHER, LAO TZU,** created this quote that we have hanging up in our kitchen. We placed it there so we can see these words and try to live by them every day:

> Watch your *thoughts* for they become words.
> Watch your *words* for they become actions.
> Watch your *actions* for they become habits.
> Watch your *habits* for they become character.
> Watch your *character* for it becomes your *destiny*.

The foundation of your emotional environment is, indeed, your thoughts and words. This is the one environment over which you have one-hundred percent complete control. Some of you may think Dr. Jill and I are fun to be around (*and most of the time we are!*). But, if you hang around us long enough you may feel like banging your head against a wall or throwing up a little because we are constantly repeating and reaffirming over and over again what we are grateful for, why we feel abundant, and what we are going to accomplish. Other mammals don't have this ability, but all humans have the freedom to think and speak for themselves. And believe me, focusing on what is *wanted* really works. These days when cool things happen to us, we've stopped being surprised. We know we deliberately created the environment that produced those results. You have the same power, and no one can take it from you, no matter what.

Keeping it real, the opposite is also true. Many people believe that when negativity comes their way, it comes out of oblivion. In fact, it came out of the oblivious. They weren't mindful of their thoughts. Their thoughts manifested into the reality in front of them. I can personally admit to some negative outcomes from sloppy thinking and misdirected energy. So, please, choose your thoughts wisely.

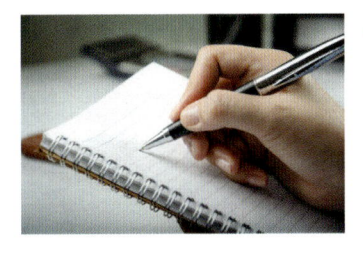

- When has sloppy thinking led to a less-than-desirable outcome in your life?

  _____
  _____
  _____

- Which thoughts usually dominate your self-talk and inner dialogue?

  _____
  _____
  _____

- When was the last time your thoughts and focus aligned with your goal and you achieved it?

  _____
  _____
  _____

# EPILOGUE

**MY GOAL IN THIS BOOK** was to give you a road map to help you prioritize your health and show you how to live your best life. I hope you follow it and reach your own personal paradise. For me, paradise is an abundance of family, friends, sunshine, joy, love, kindness, laughter, inner peace, overall well-being, and a feeling of unlimited potential.

I want to reiterate what I wrote at the beginning of the book as I leave you with my final thoughts. Remember, no matter what happened to you, whether it was an injury, crisis, or setback, you can either be a victim or a survivor. In order to survive and advance, endure and conquer, or move onwards and upwards, you need to prioritize your health. When it comes to living your best life, if you have your health, you have hope. If you have hope, you have everything.

Onwards and upwards!

*Marcello*

# INSPIRATION

*"Photography is an art of observation. It has little to do with the things you see and everything to do with how you see them."*

—ELLIOT ERWIT

**I REALLY ENJOY PHOTOGRAPHY.** I pride myself on seeing things in a positive light. I like to observe people, interesting things, and scenic landscapes. I appreciate beauty in all forms. I also love to inspire and empower my family, friends, and clients. Although some images are forever etched in my mind, I tend to forget a lot of things that cross my path after I see them. Taking pictures and pairing them with some of my favorite quotes not only helps me remember awesome experiences and moments, but it has also turned out to be quite a delightful and productive use of my time and energy. The following section features a sampling of my "Enjoy Your Weekend" inspirational memes that I post online on Friday mornings. The first collection that I compiled for *Celebrate Life* was well-received, so I hope you enjoy this gallery of "Inspo-memes" as well.

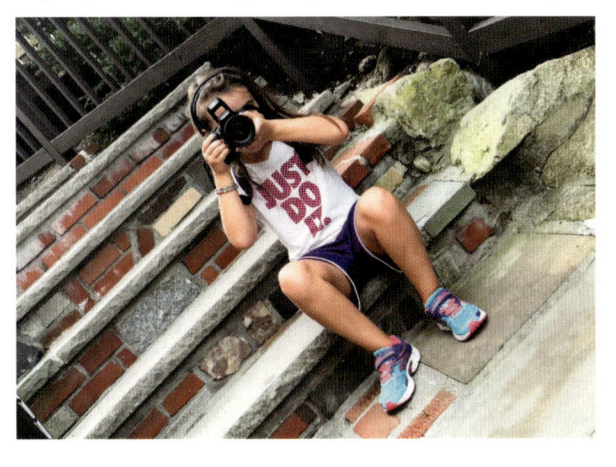

*"It's never too late. For with a purpose, a worthy goal, and a motivation to reach those upper layers on the pyramid, a person can travel further in a few years than he might otherwise travel in a lifetime."*
~Earl Nightingale

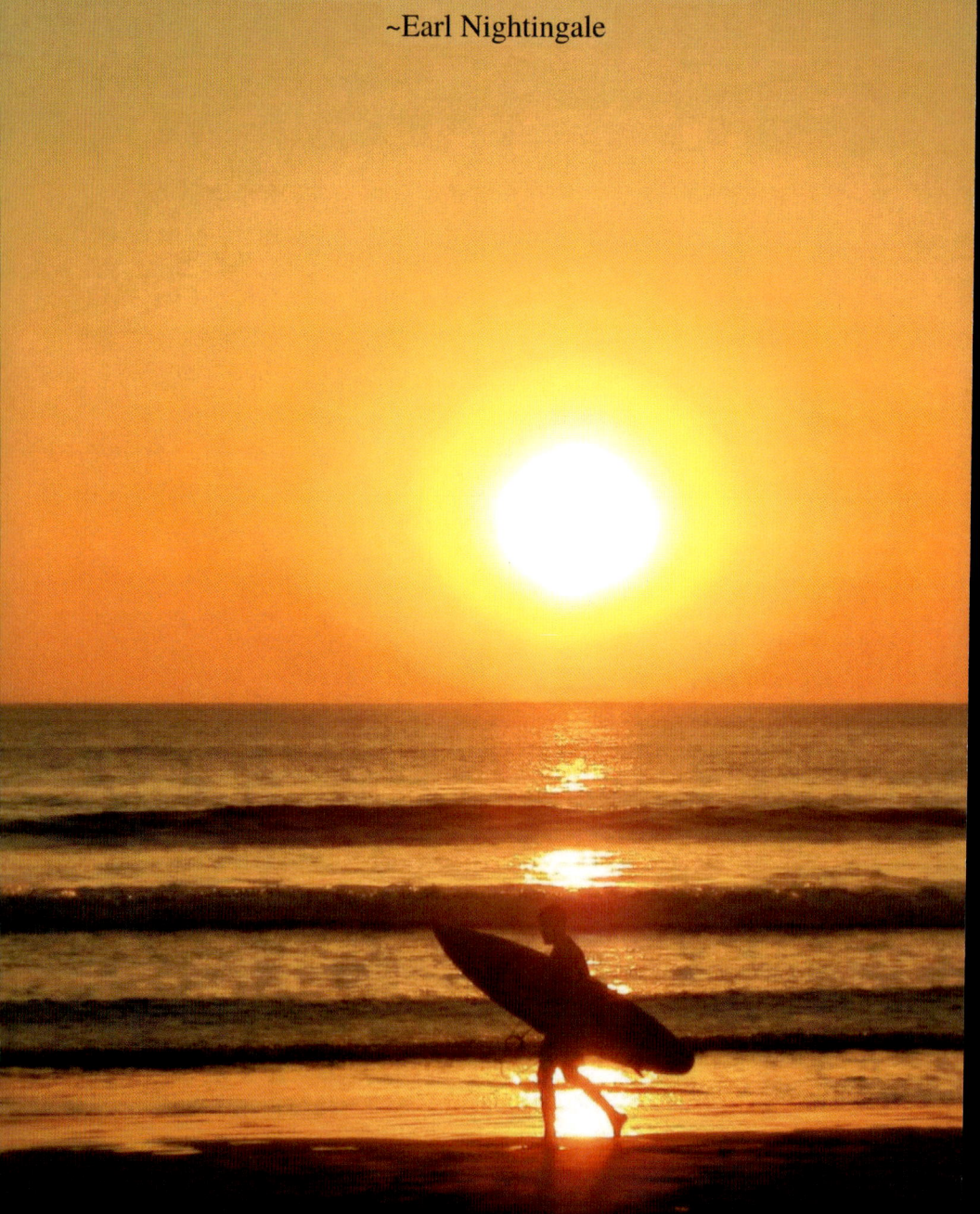

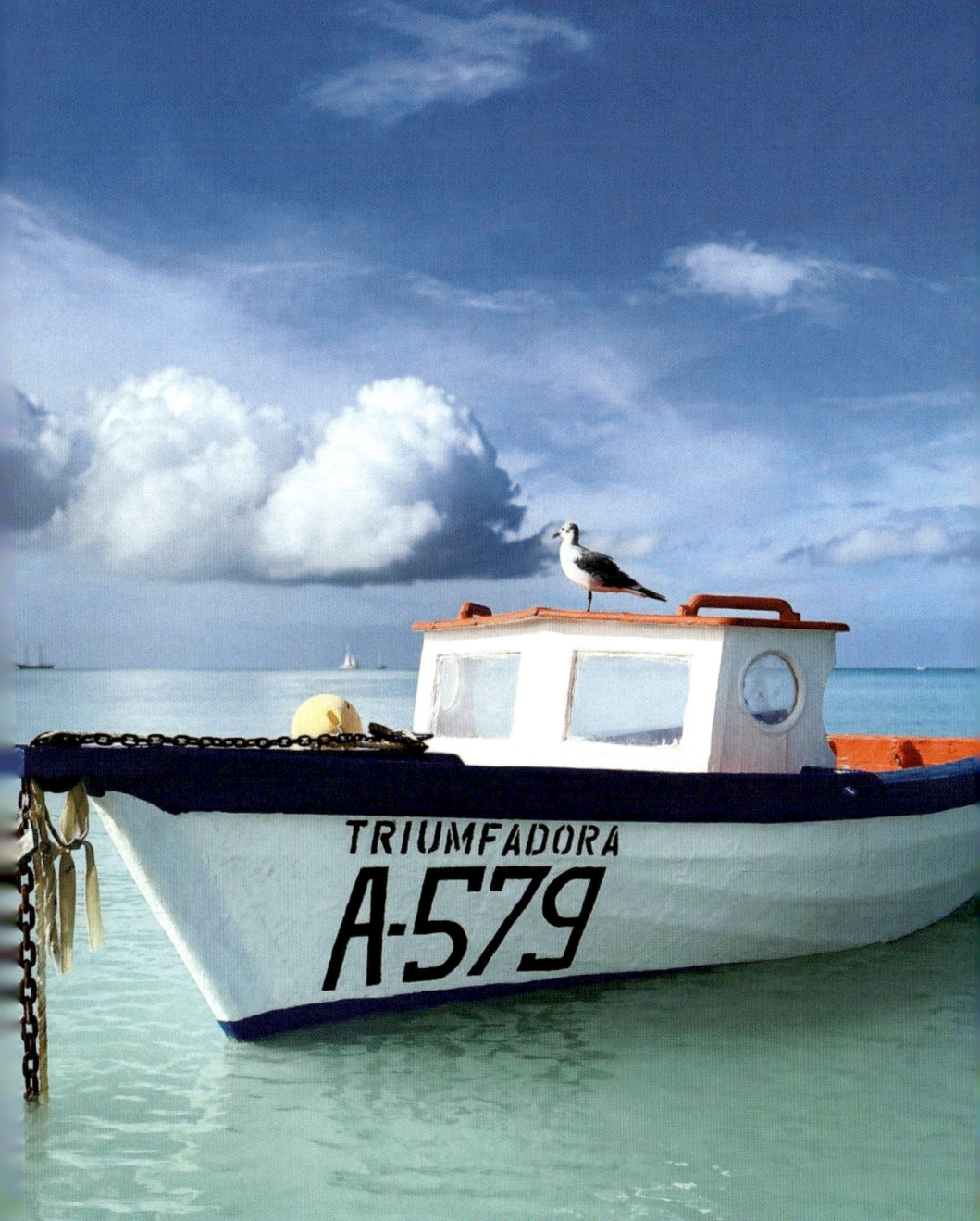

"We lose ourselves in the things we love.
We find ourselves there, too."
~Kristin Martz

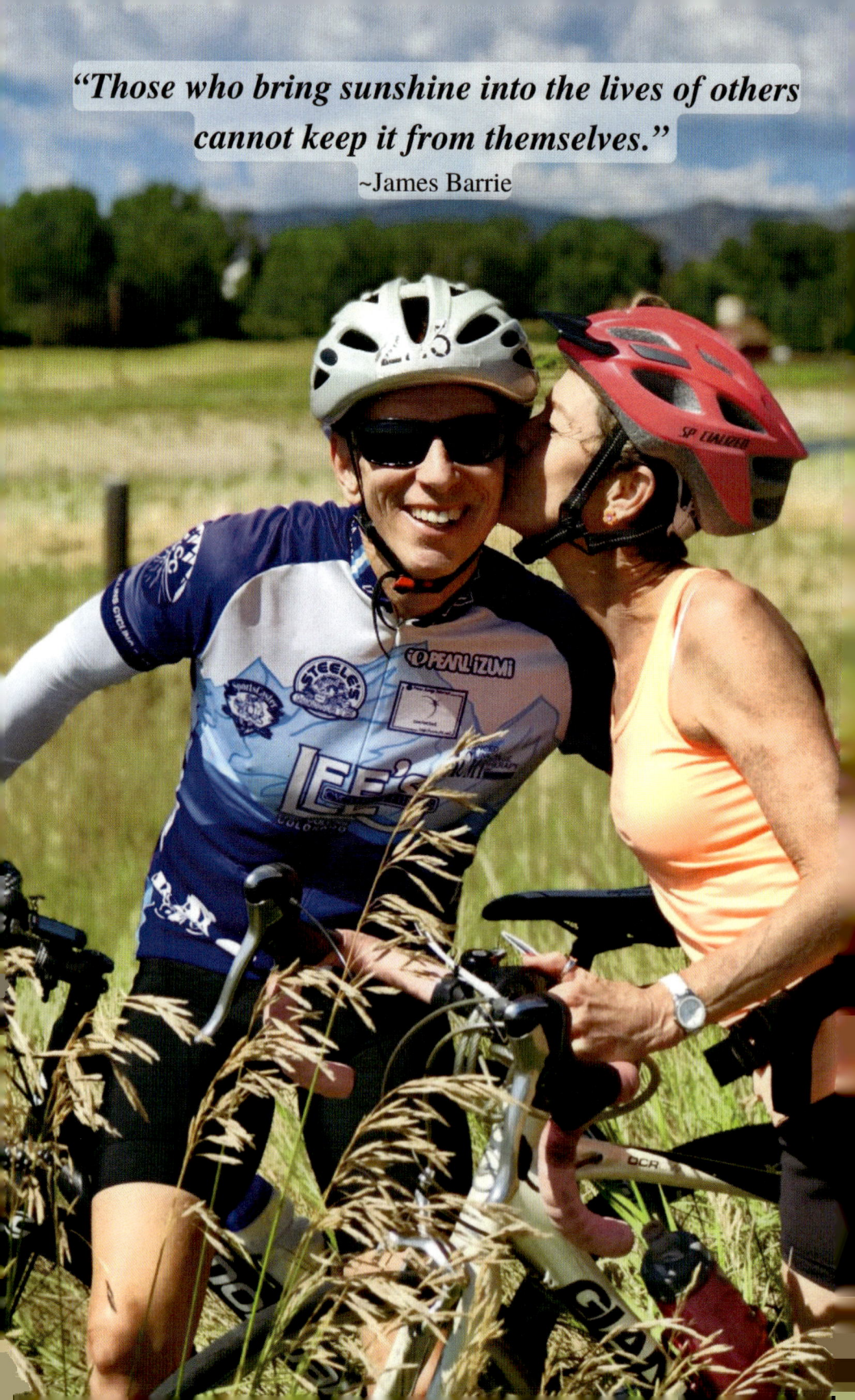

*"Those who bring sunshine into the lives of others cannot keep it from themselves."*
~James Barrie

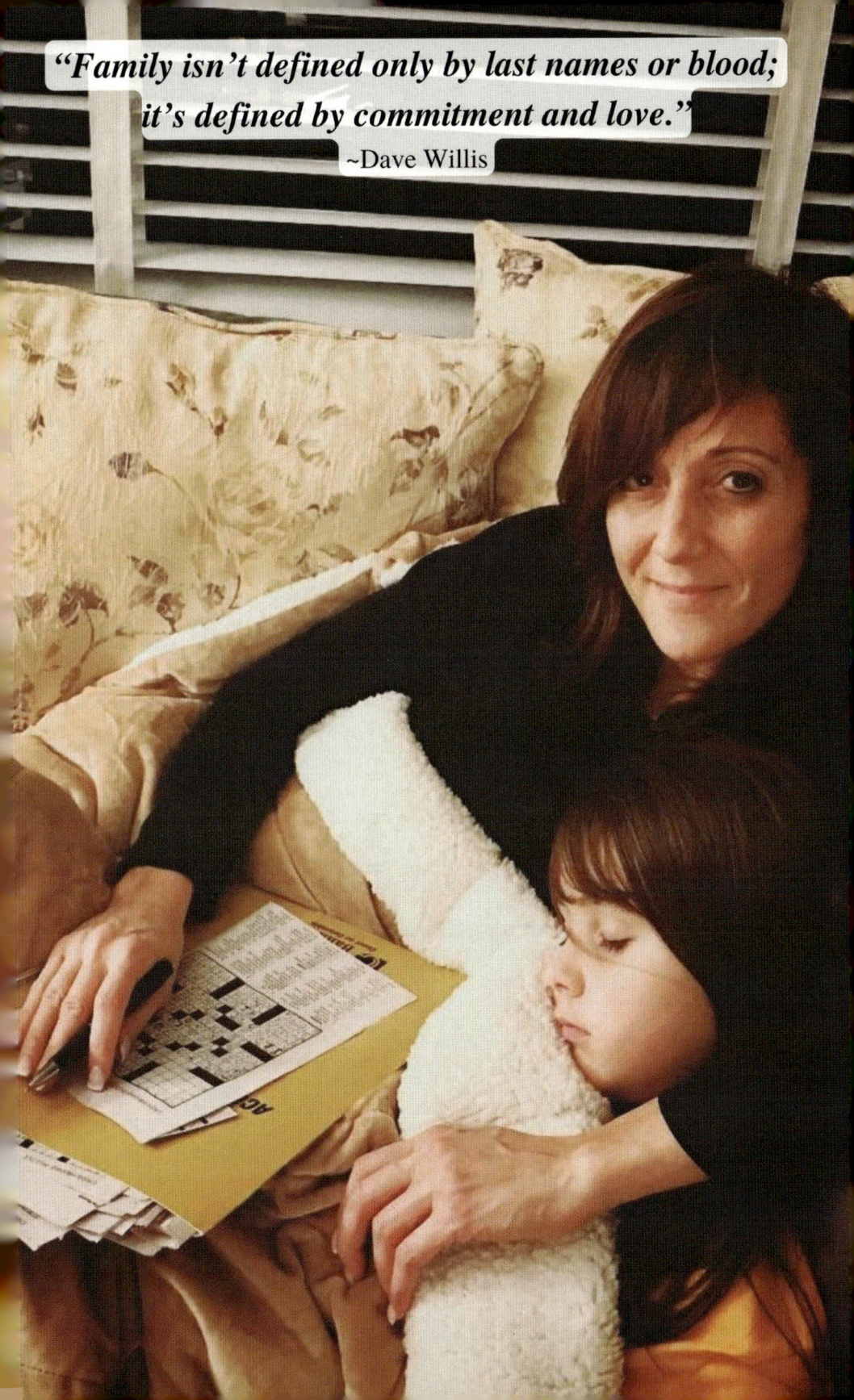

"Family isn't defined only by last names or blood; it's defined by commitment and love."
~Dave Willis

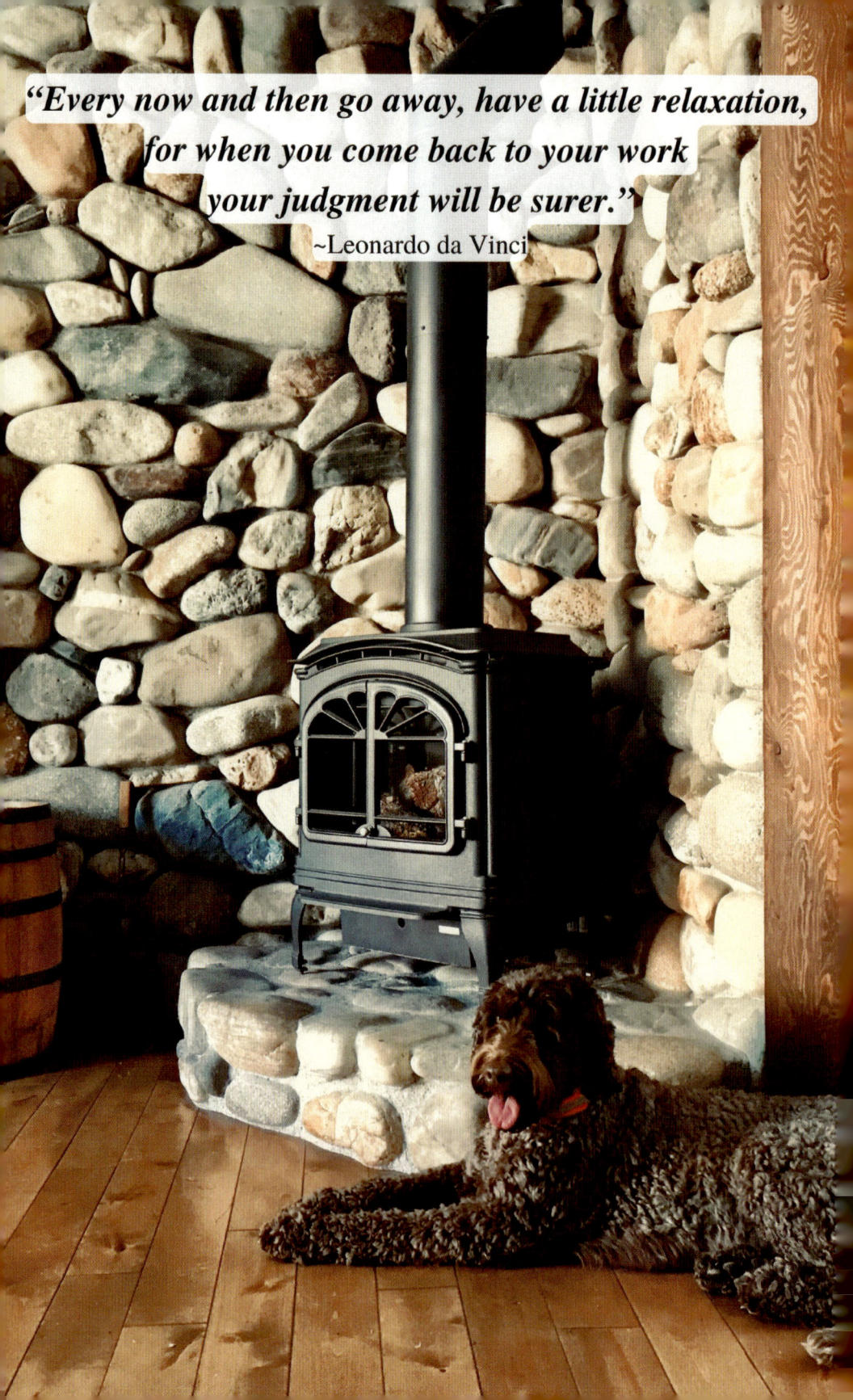

*"Every now and then go away, have a little relaxation, for when you come back to your work your judgment will be surer."*
~Leonardo da Vinci

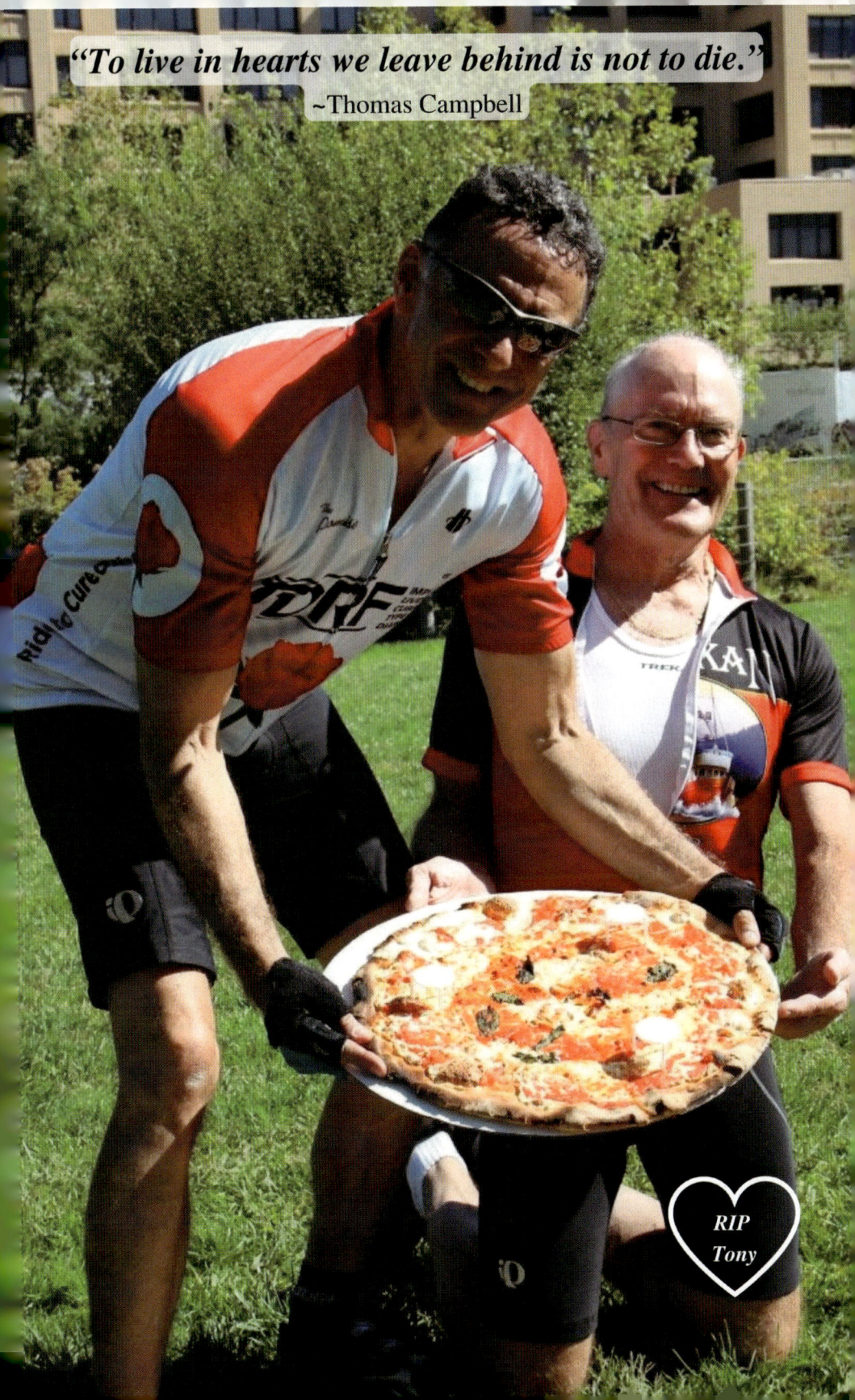

*"To live in hearts we leave behind is not to die."*
~Thomas Campbell

*RIP Tony*

"Ask yourself how many people you know are living with any real understanding of the crazy locomotive called life. Most people are passive pawns in the ride, clueless how th machinery works, the source of its octane, how to manage its direction, or its velocity, or, above all, who their chauffe is. They talk of free will, liberty, and independence but the have little or no control over their lives. Their destiny is something they create unconsciously.
Welcome to Karma, a dimension that puts you squarely back where you belong along: in the driver's seat."

~Sadhguru

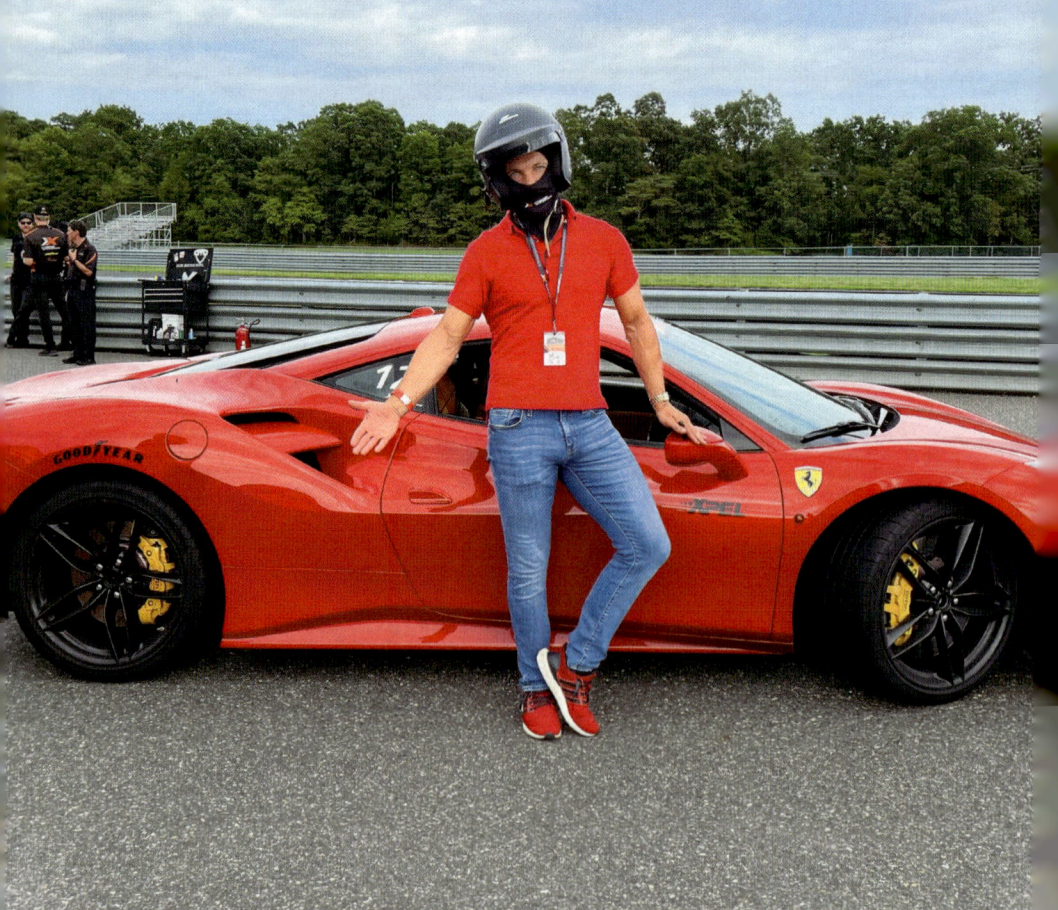

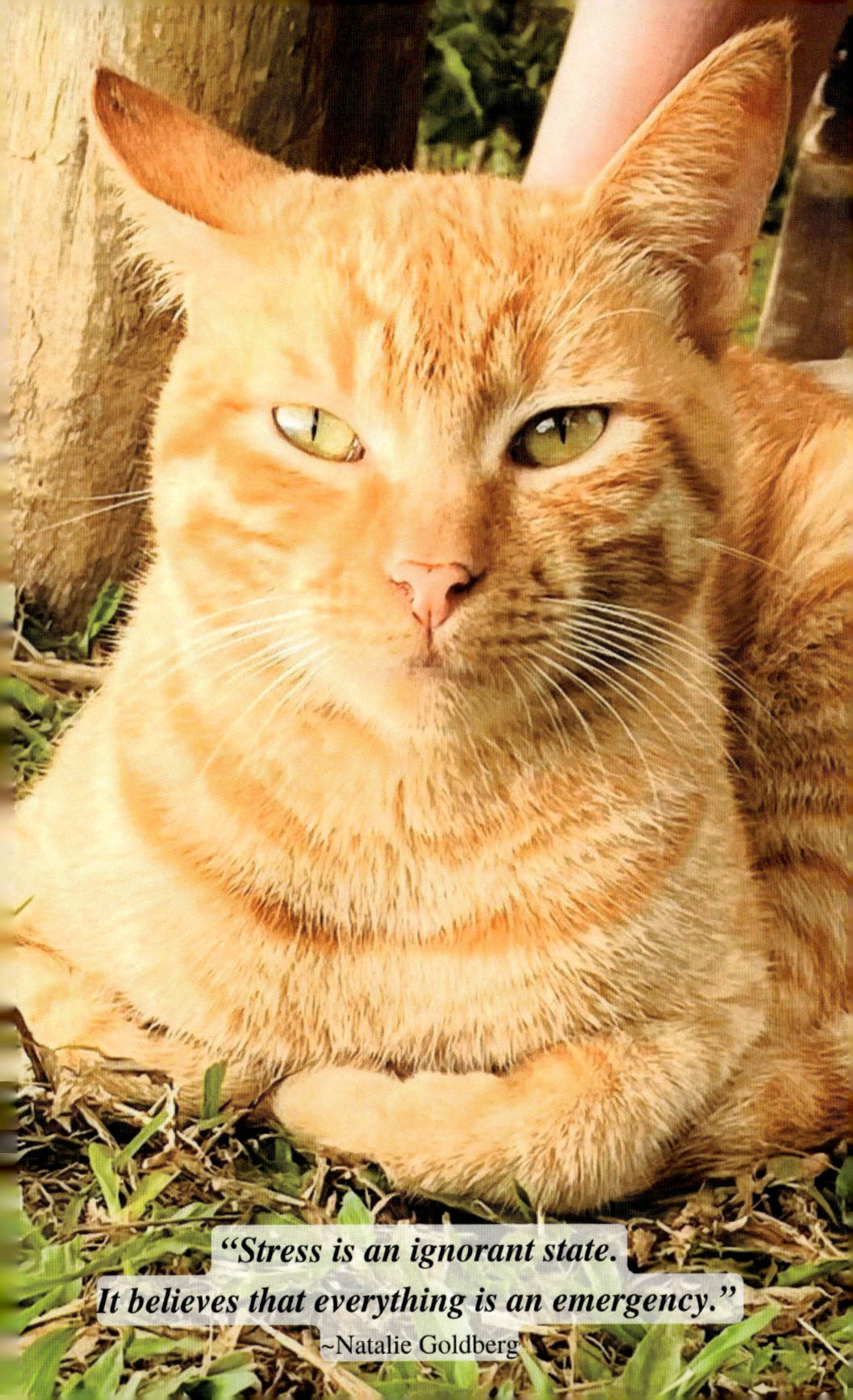

"Stress is an ignorant state.
It believes that everything is an emergency."
~Natalie Goldberg

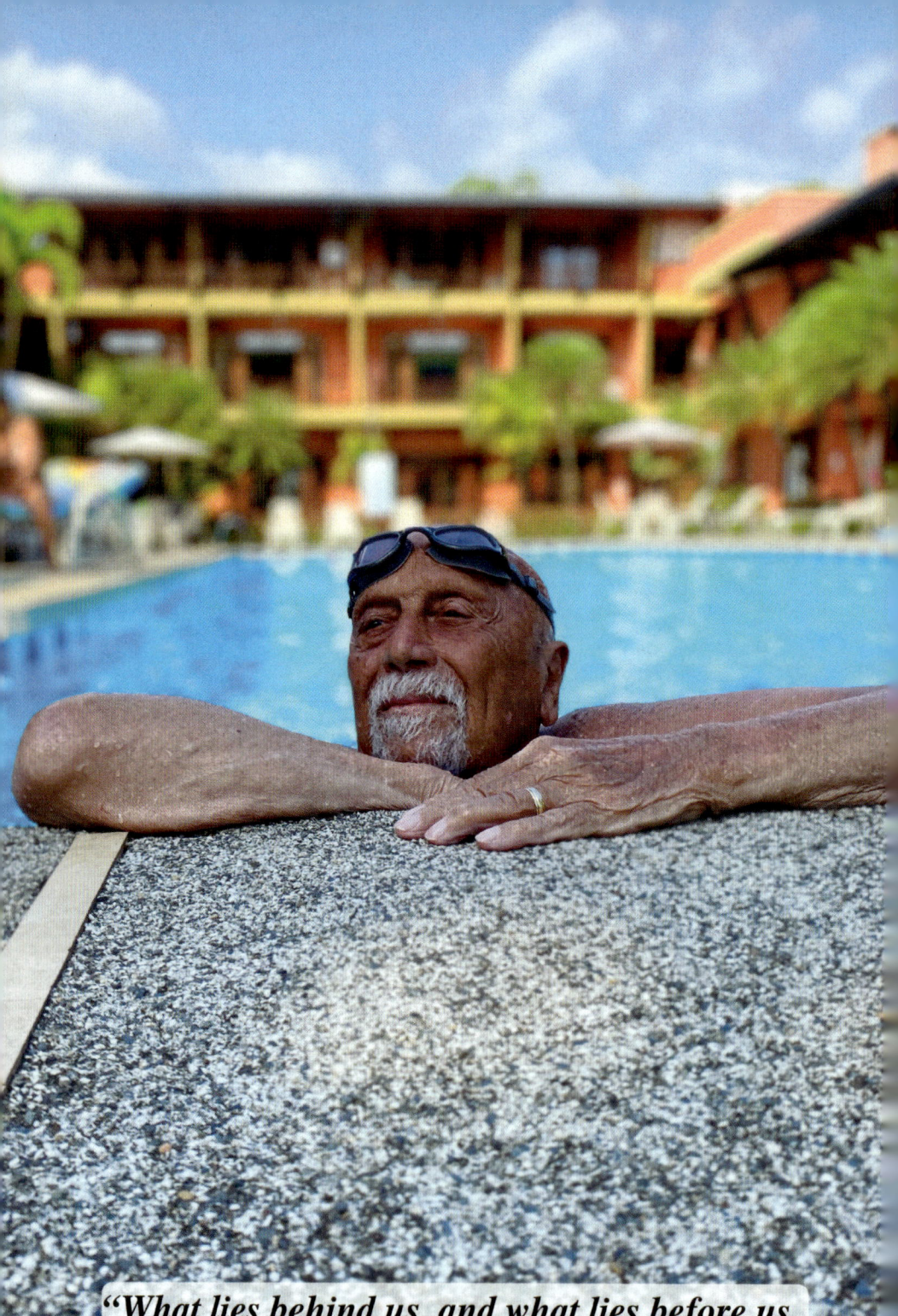

"What lies behind us, and what lies before us, are tiny matters compared to what lies within us."
~Ralph Waldo Emerson

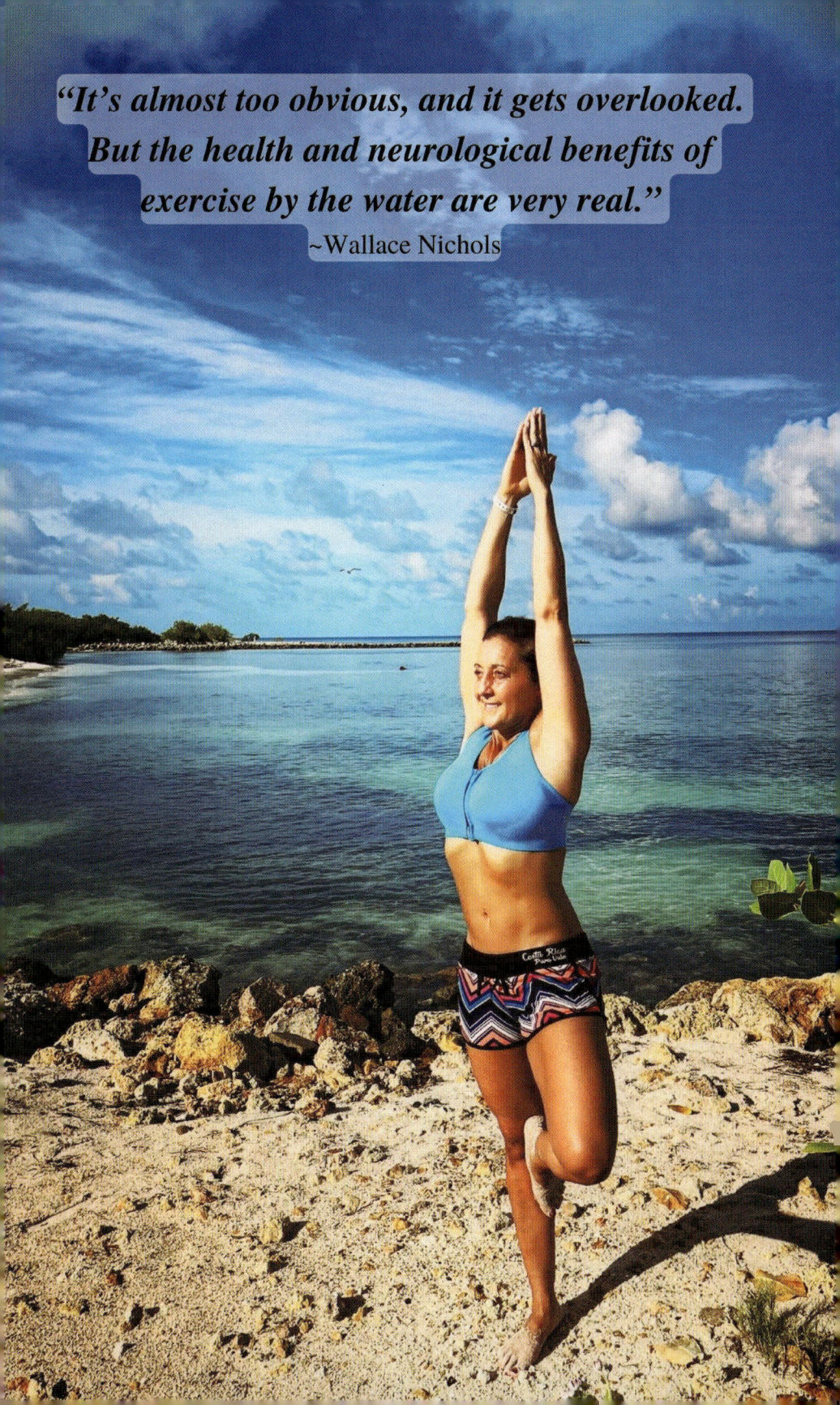

> "It's almost too obvious, and it gets overlooked. But the health and neurological benefits of exercise by the water are very real."
> ~Wallace Nichols

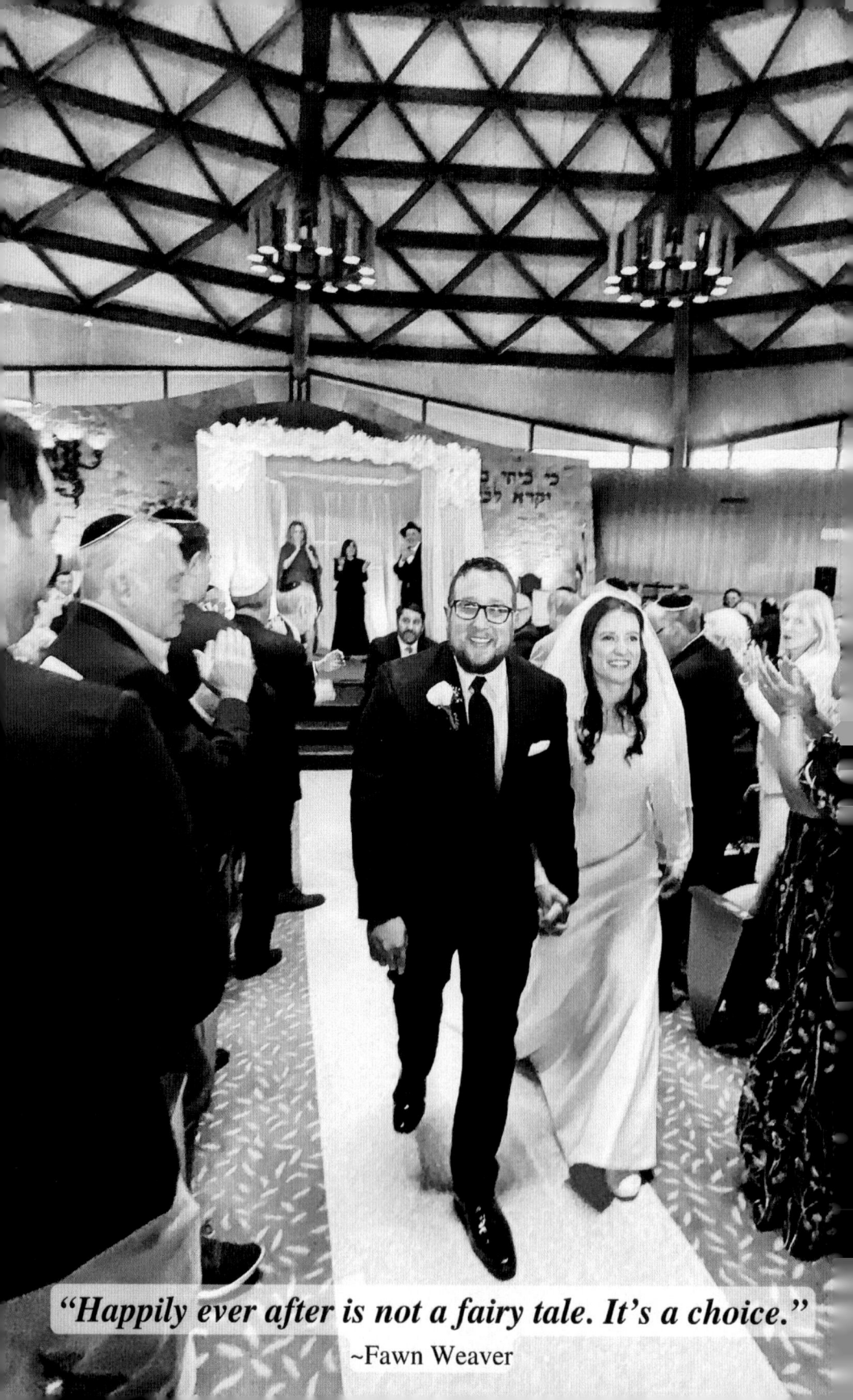

"Happily ever after is not a fairy tale. It's a choice."
~Fawn Weaver

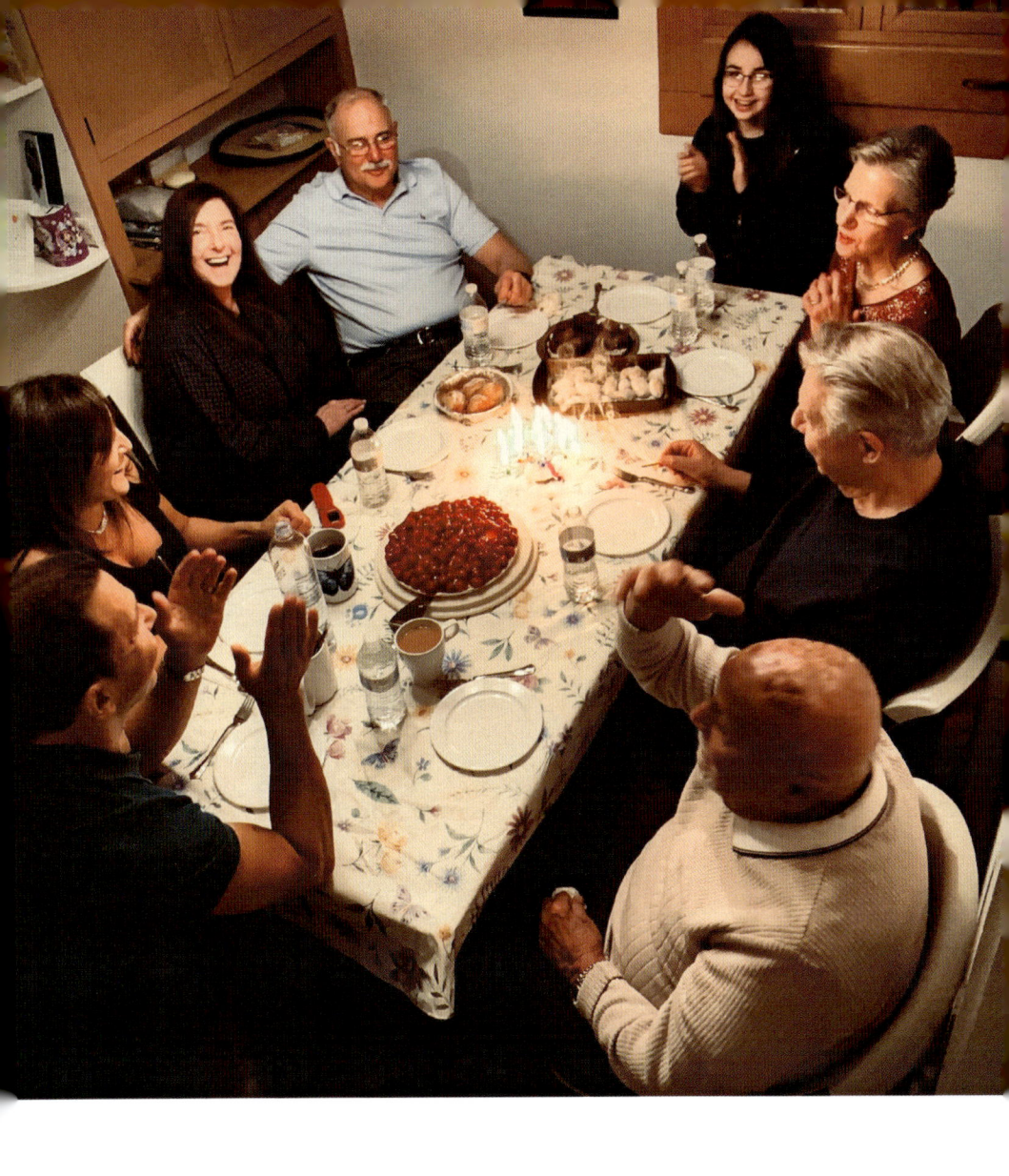

*"A dining table… with the eager faces of those we love gathered around it, becomes more than just a place to eat. It becomes an alter of affirmation, joy, and rest from the outside world."*

~via Jill Michaels

*"Always remember to take your Vitamins: Take your Vitamin A for Action, Vitamin B for Belief, Vitamin C for Confidence, Vitamin D for Discipline, and Vitamin E for Enthusiasm!"*
~Henry Thoreau

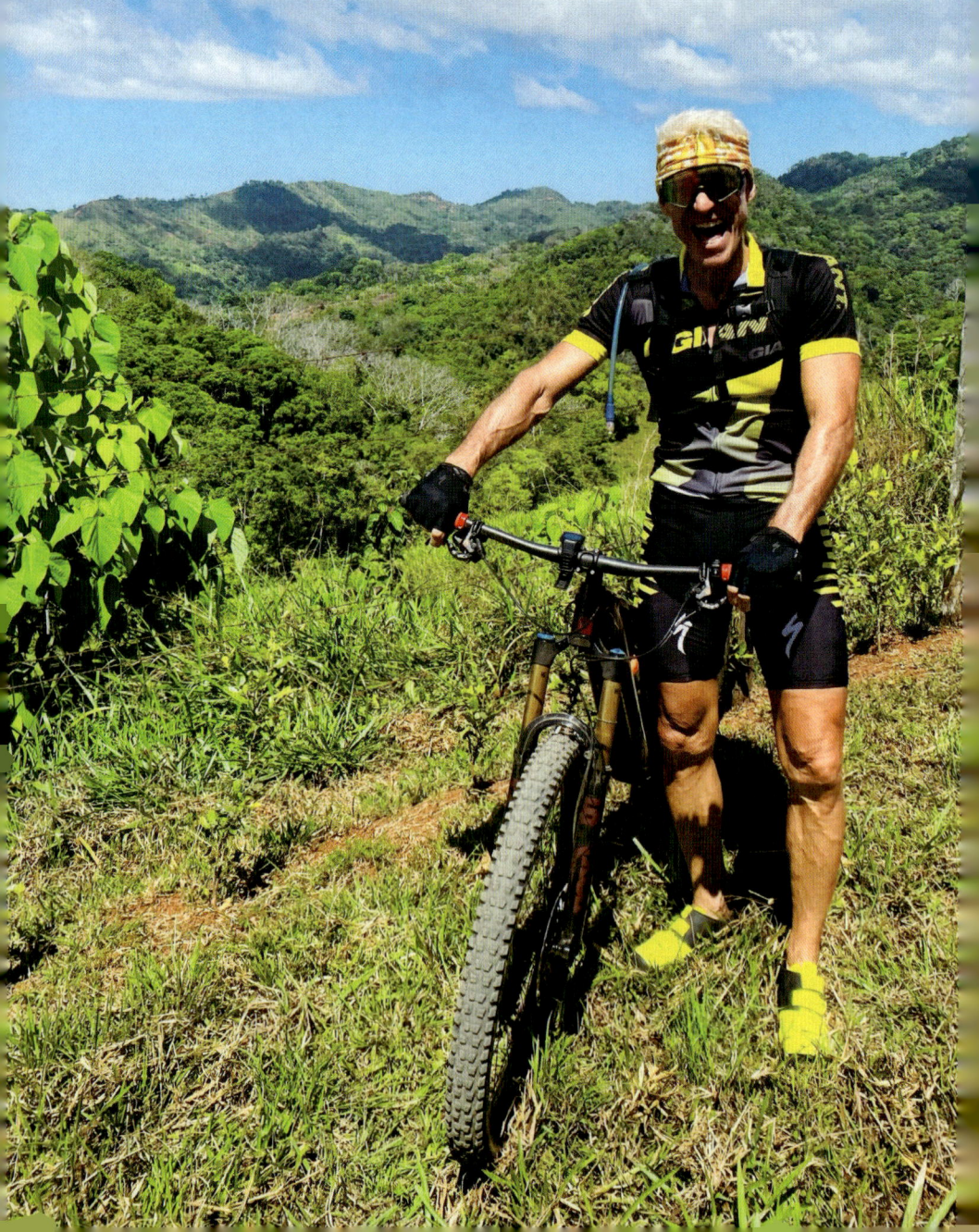

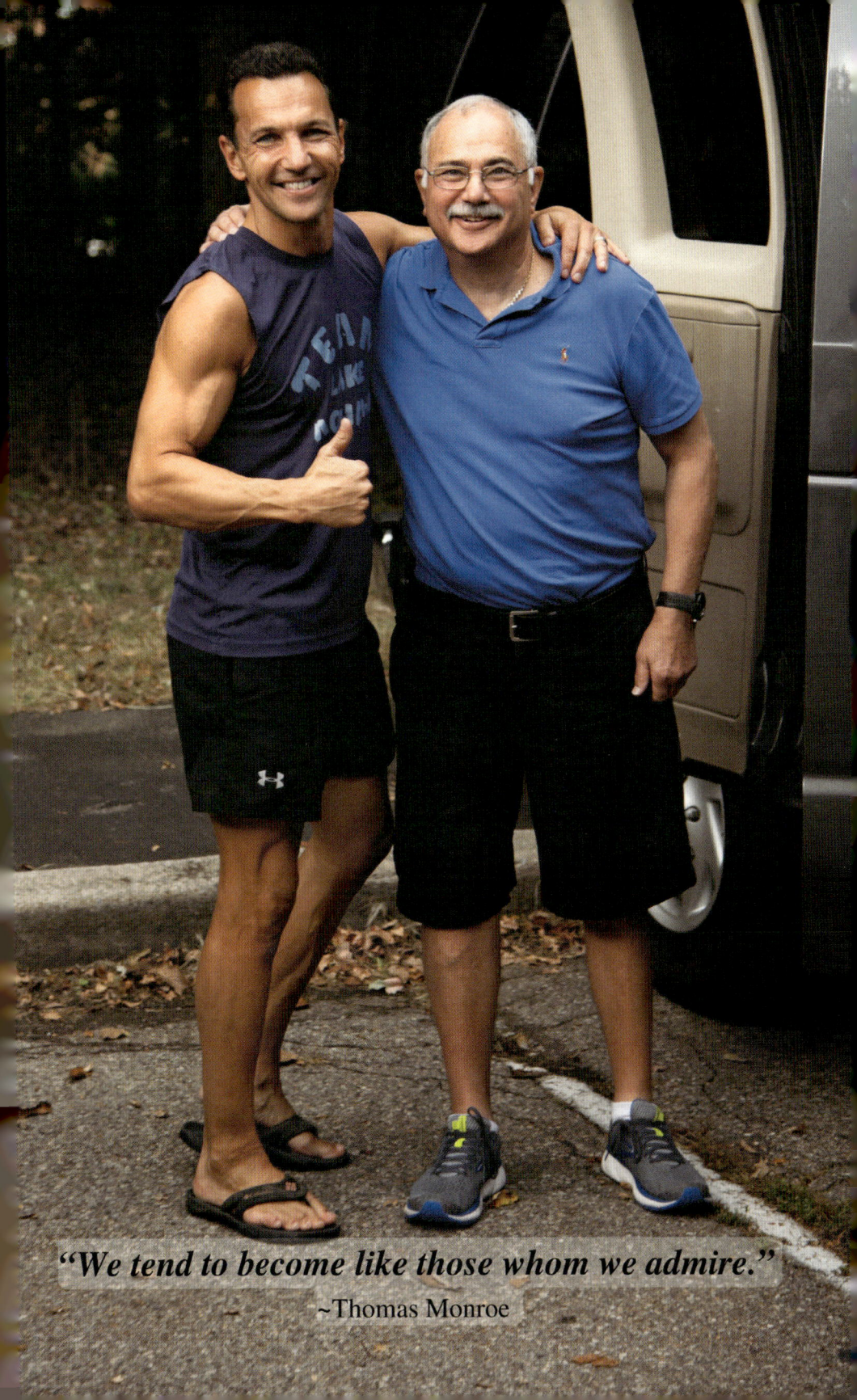

*"We tend to become like those whom we admire."*
~Thomas Monroe

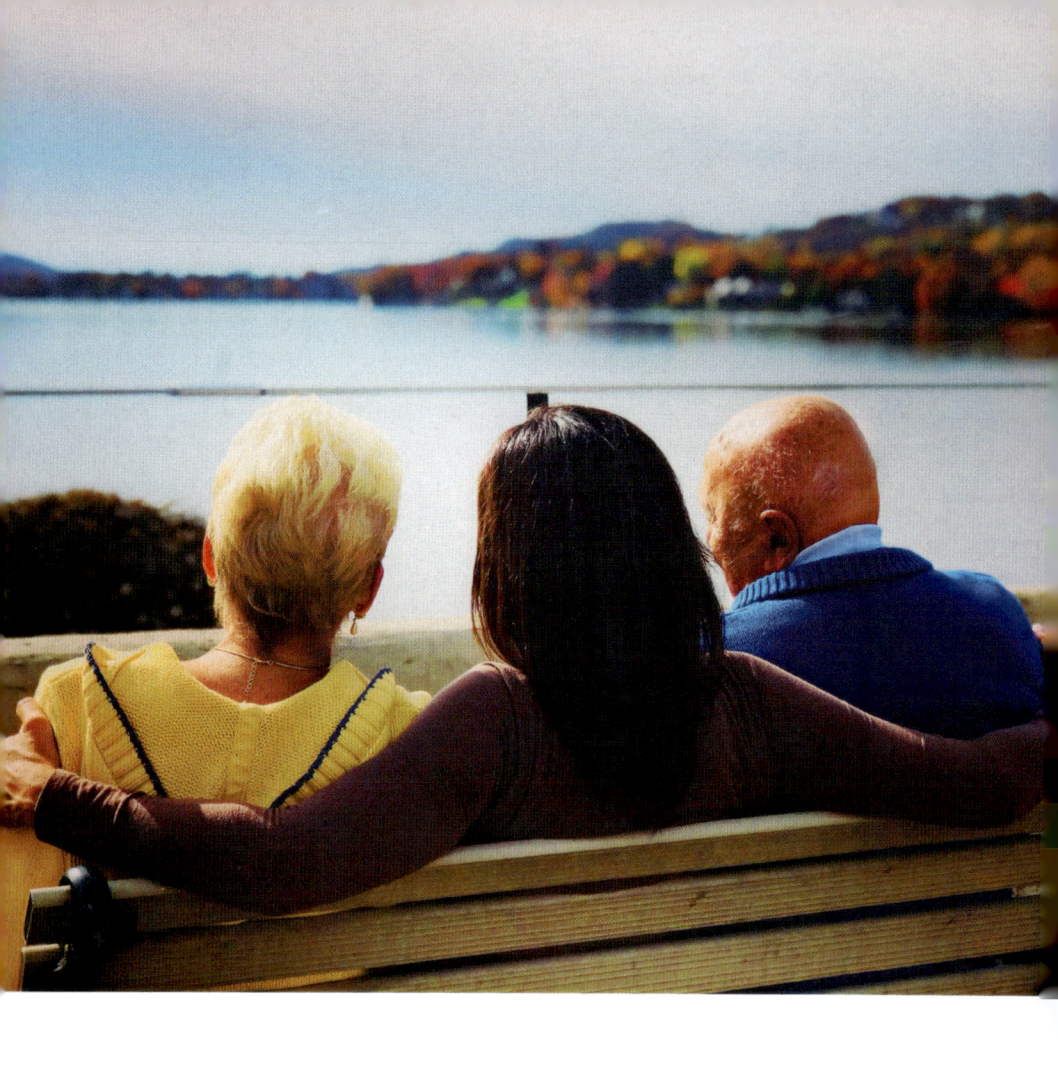

*"The family is one of nature's masterpieces."*
~George Santayana

"Life is all about balance.
Be kind, but don't let people abuse you.
Trust, but don't be deceived.
Be content, but never stop improving yourself."
~Zig Ziglar

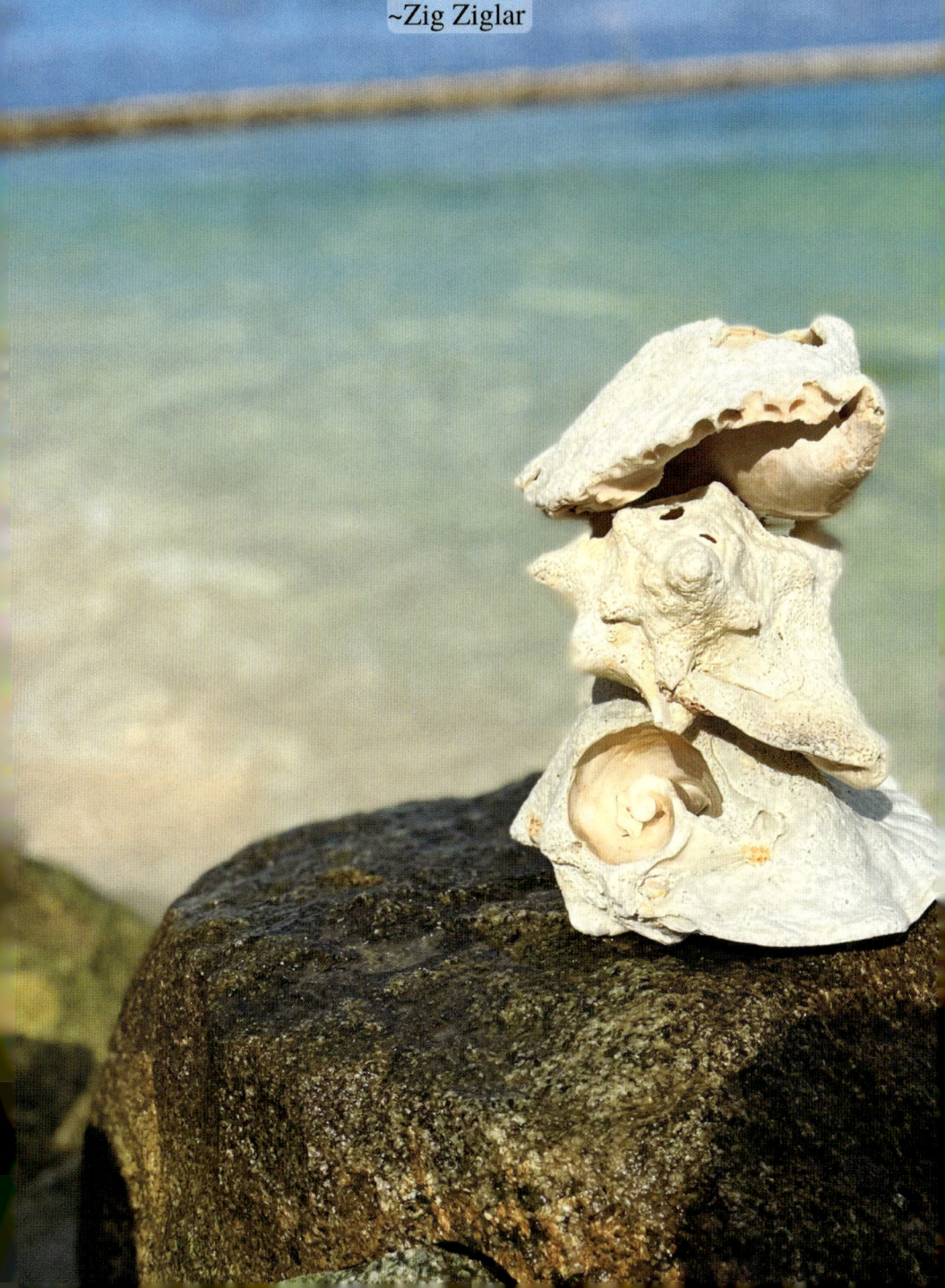

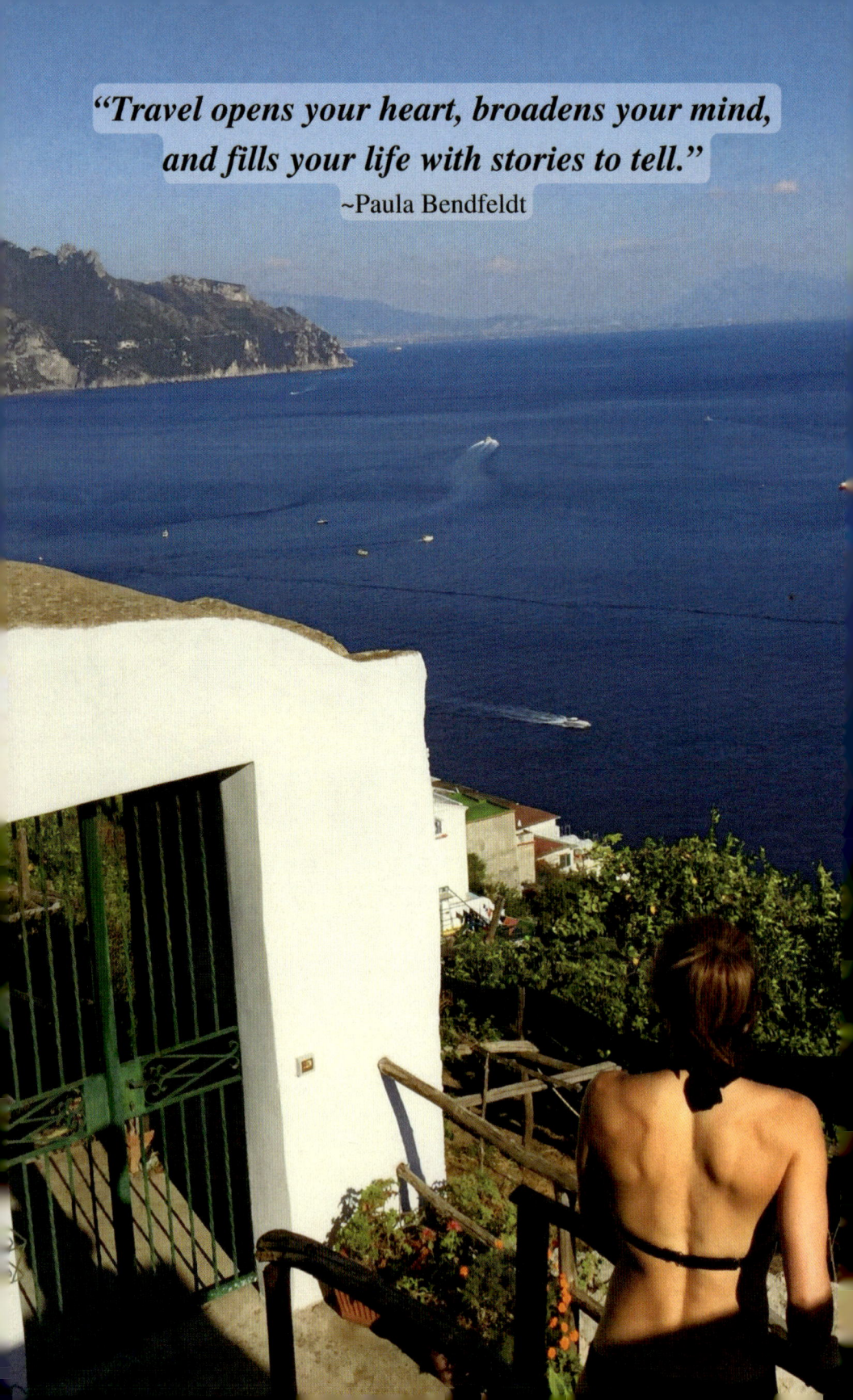

"Travel opens your heart, broadens your mind, and fills your life with stories to tell."
~Paula Bendfeldt

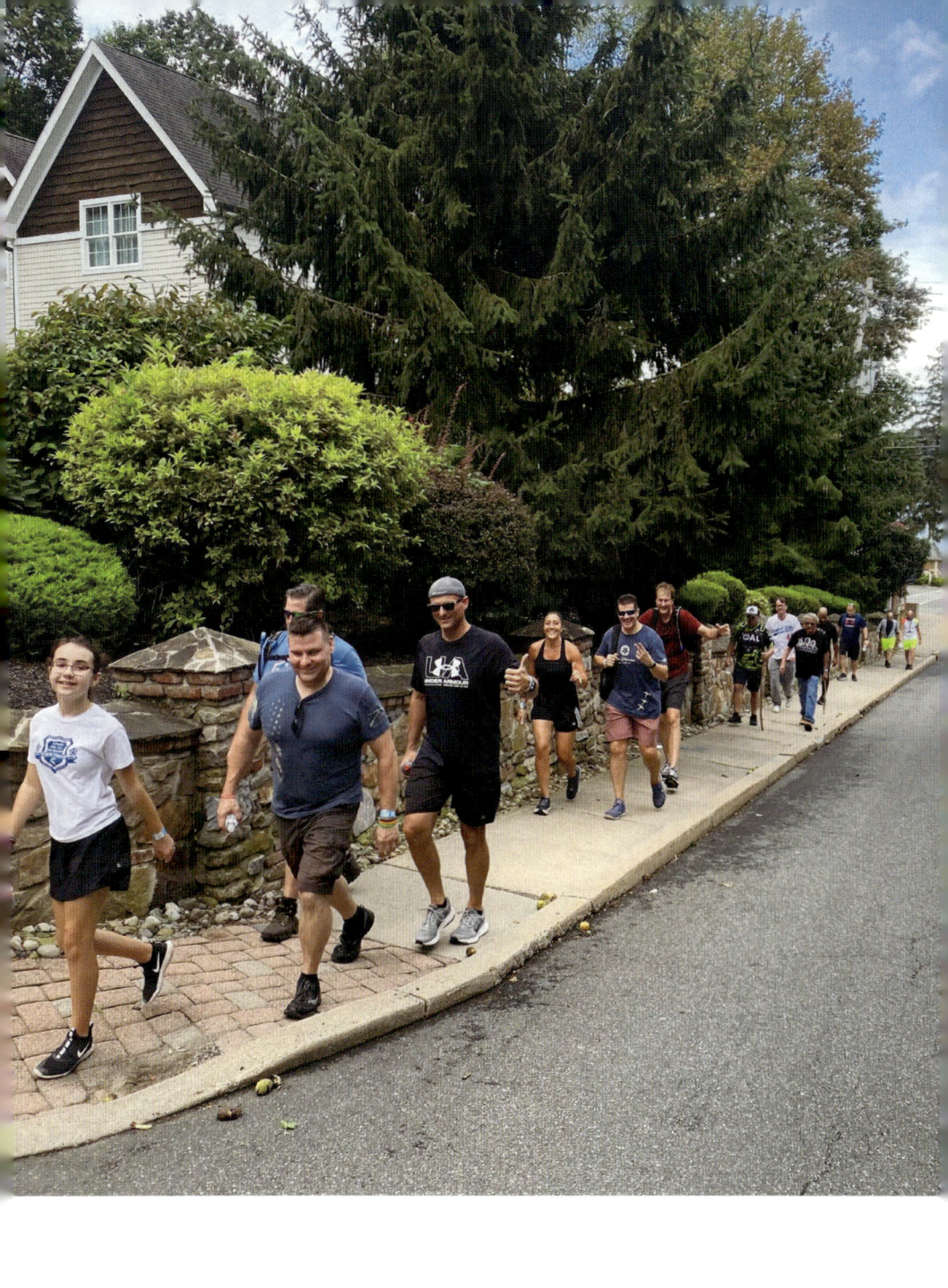

"Leadership isn't about winning.
It's about bringing people with you to the finish line."
~John Maxwell

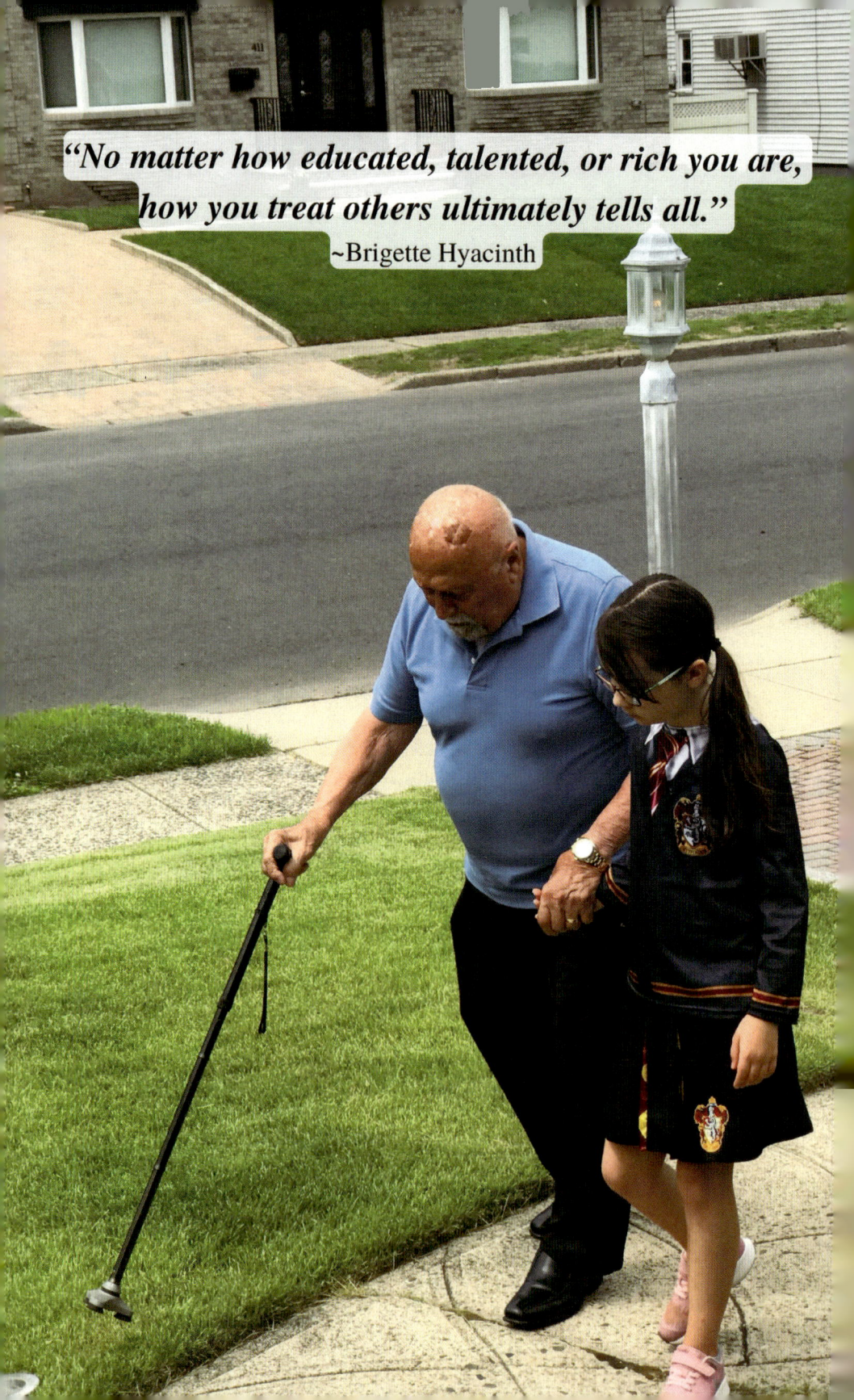

"No matter how educated, talented, or rich you are, how you treat others ultimately tells all."
~Brigette Hyacinth

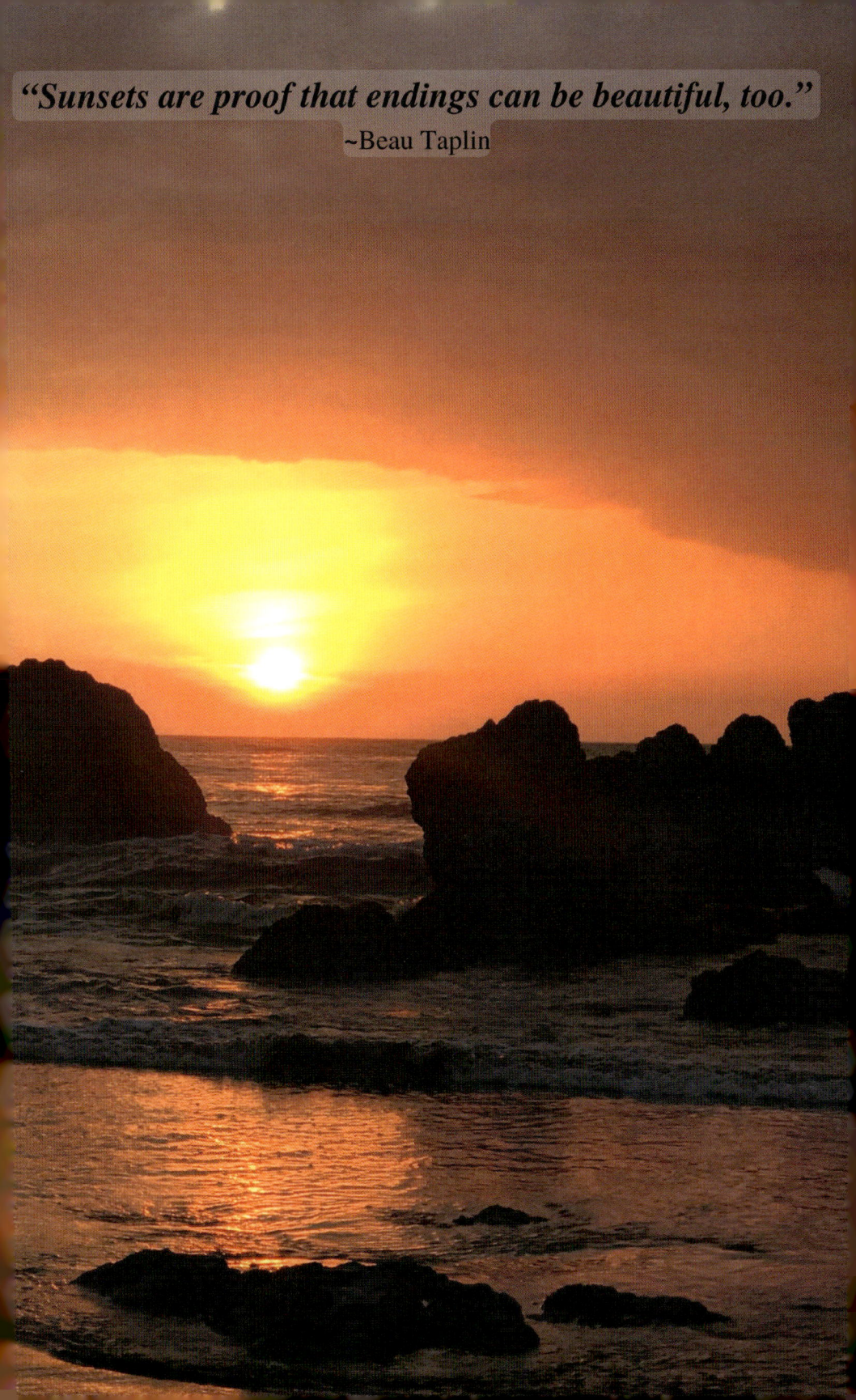

*"Sunsets are proof that endings can be beautiful, too."*
~Beau Taplin

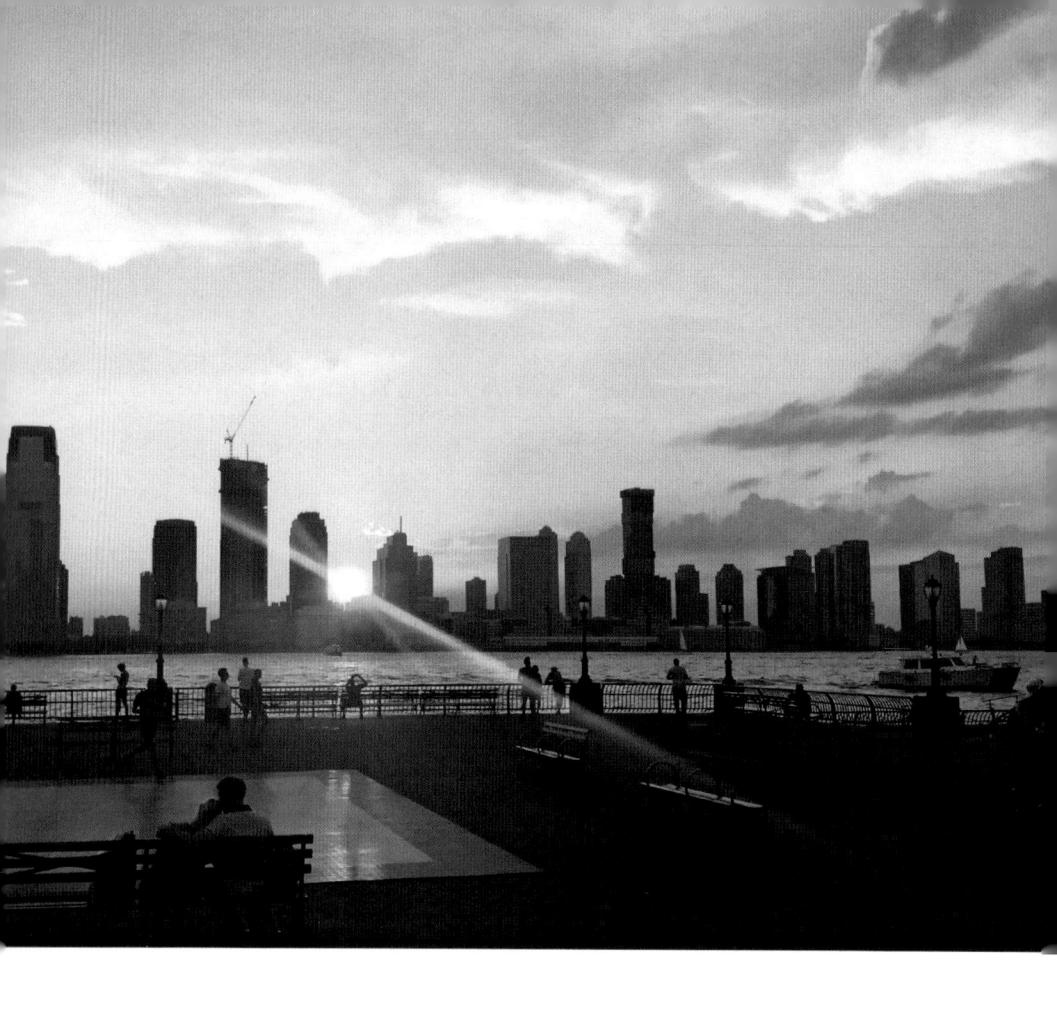

*"You can design and create, and build
the most wonderful place in the world.
But it takes people to make the dream a reality."*
~Walt Disney

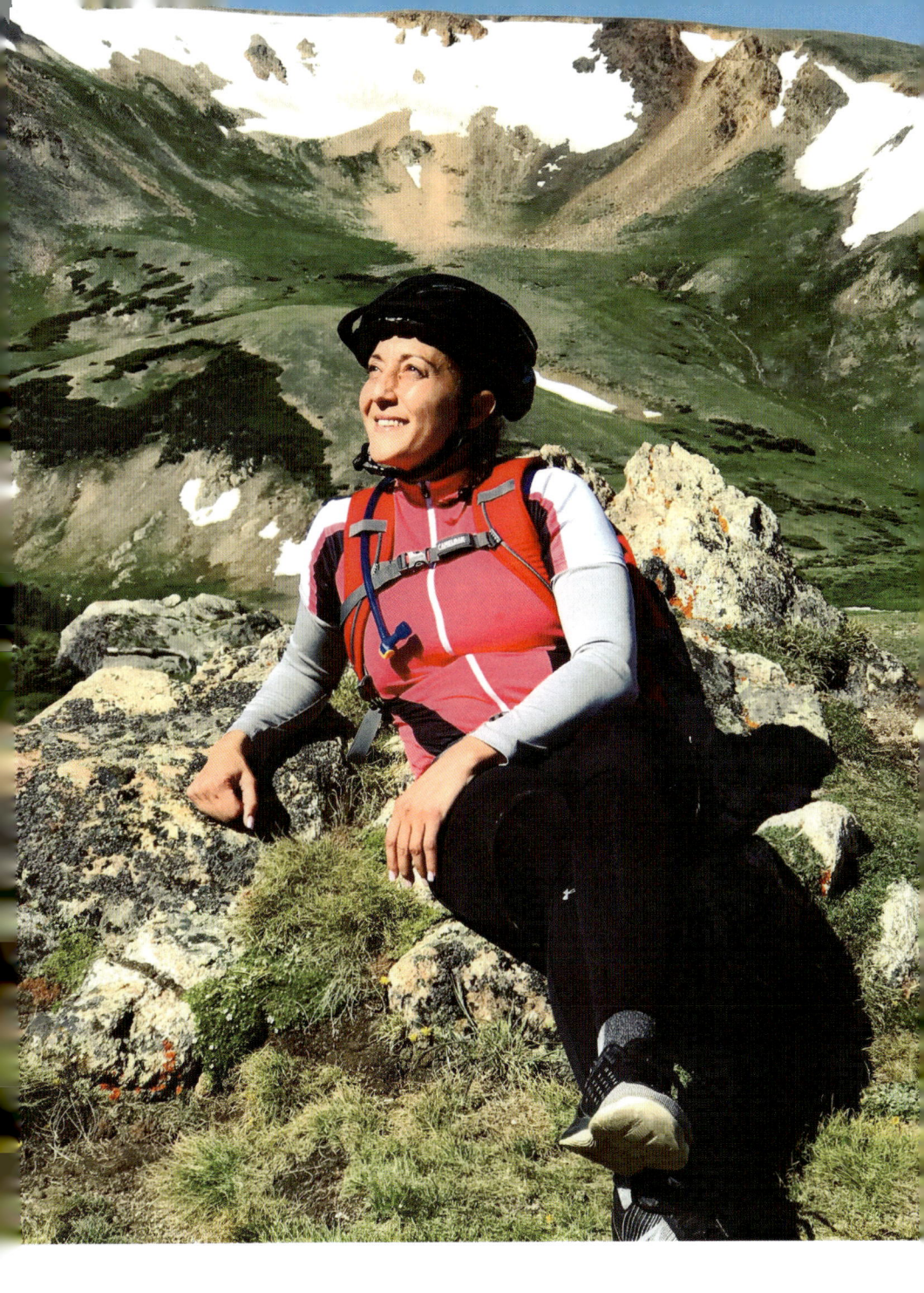

"Once in awhile, it really hits people that they don't have to experience the world in the way they've been told to."

~Alan Keightly

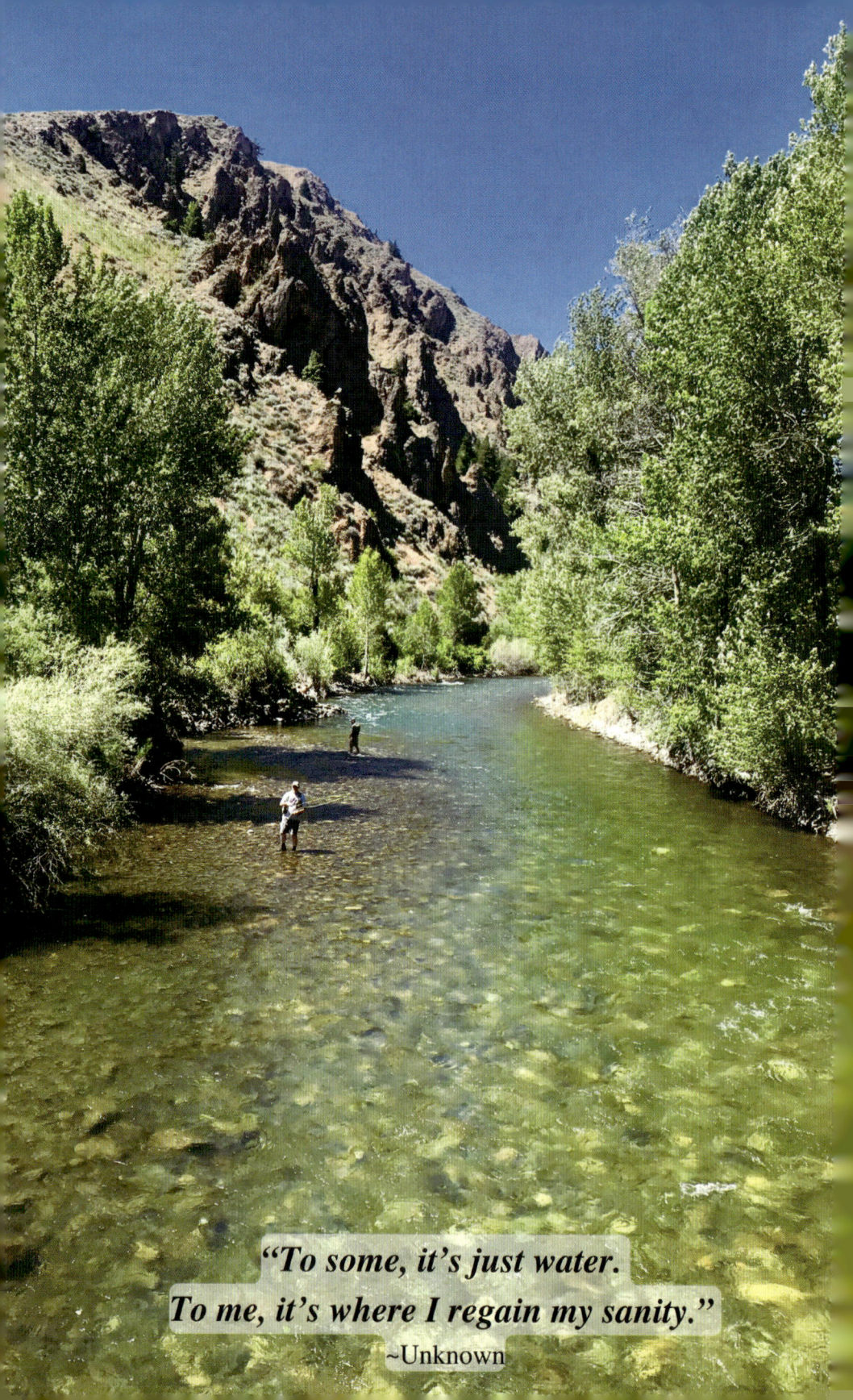

"To some, it's just water.
To me, it's where I regain my sanity."
~Unknown

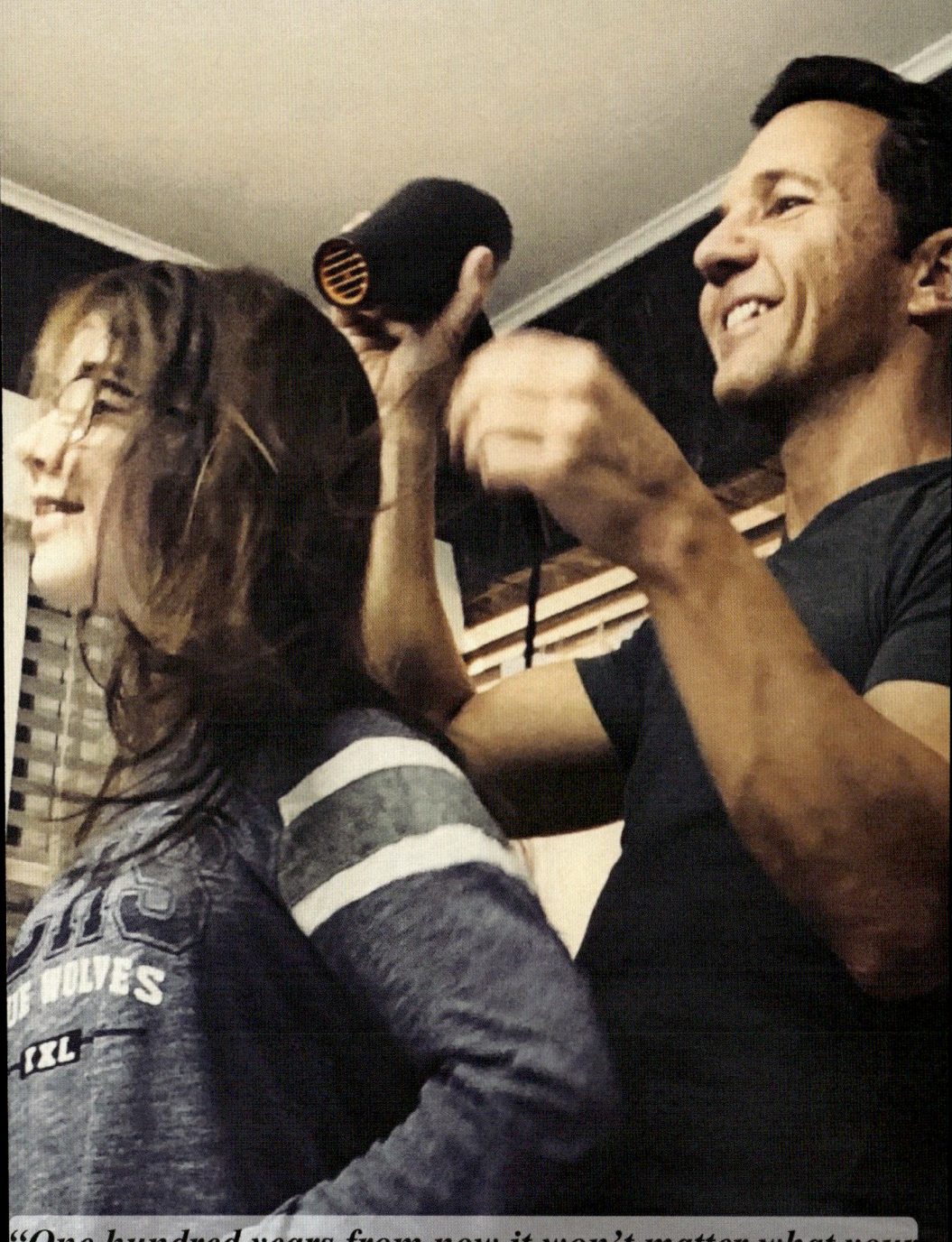

"One hundred years from now it won't matter what your bank account was, the sort of house you lived in, or the kind of car you drove, but the world may be different because you were important in the life of a child."

~Forest Whitcraft

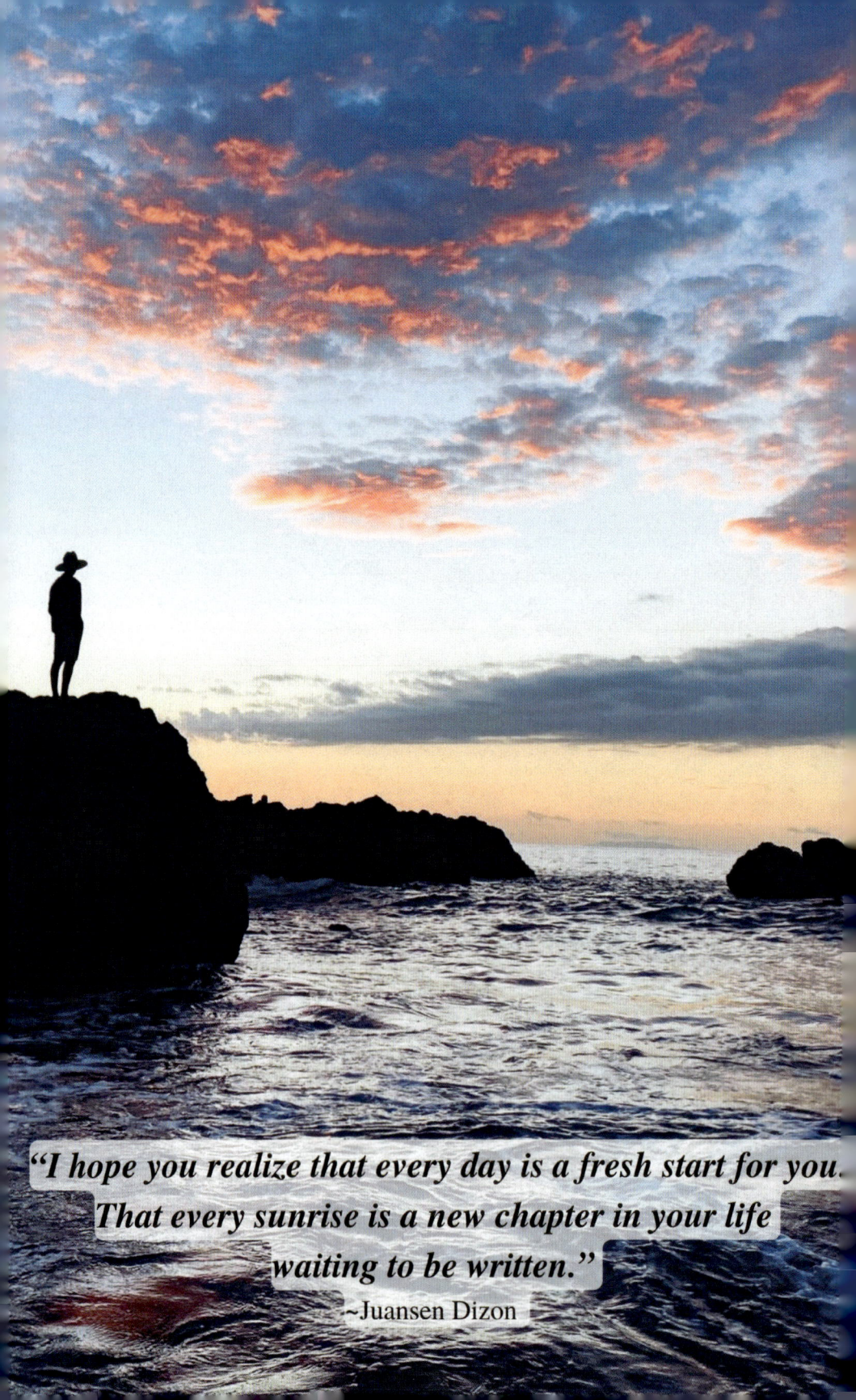

"I hope you realize that every day is a fresh start for you. That every sunrise is a new chapter in your life waiting to be written."

~Juansen Dizon

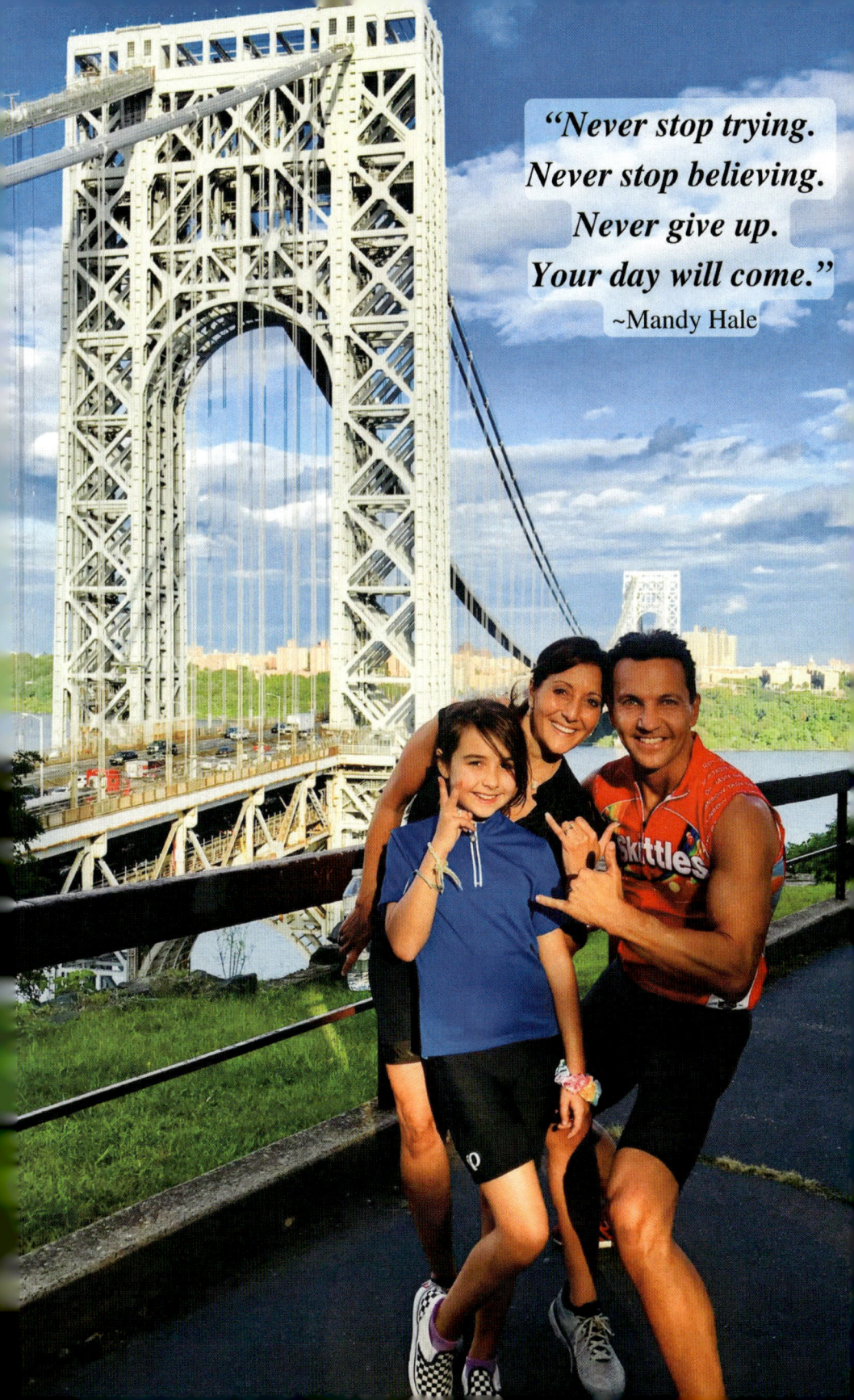

*"Never stop trying.
Never stop believing.
Never give up.
Your day will come."*
~Mandy Hale

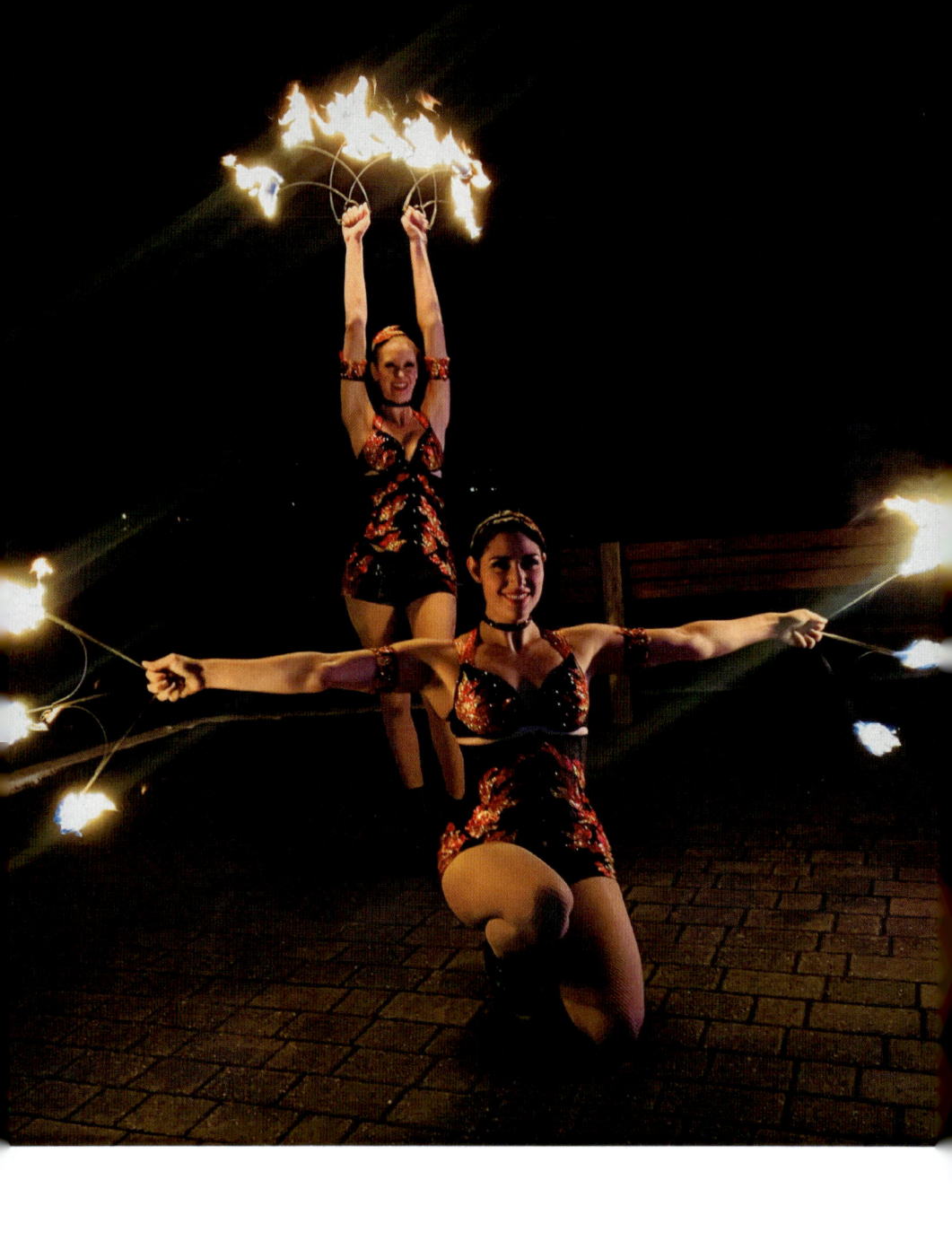

*"The happiest people are those who use their natural talents to the utmost."*
~Harv Eker

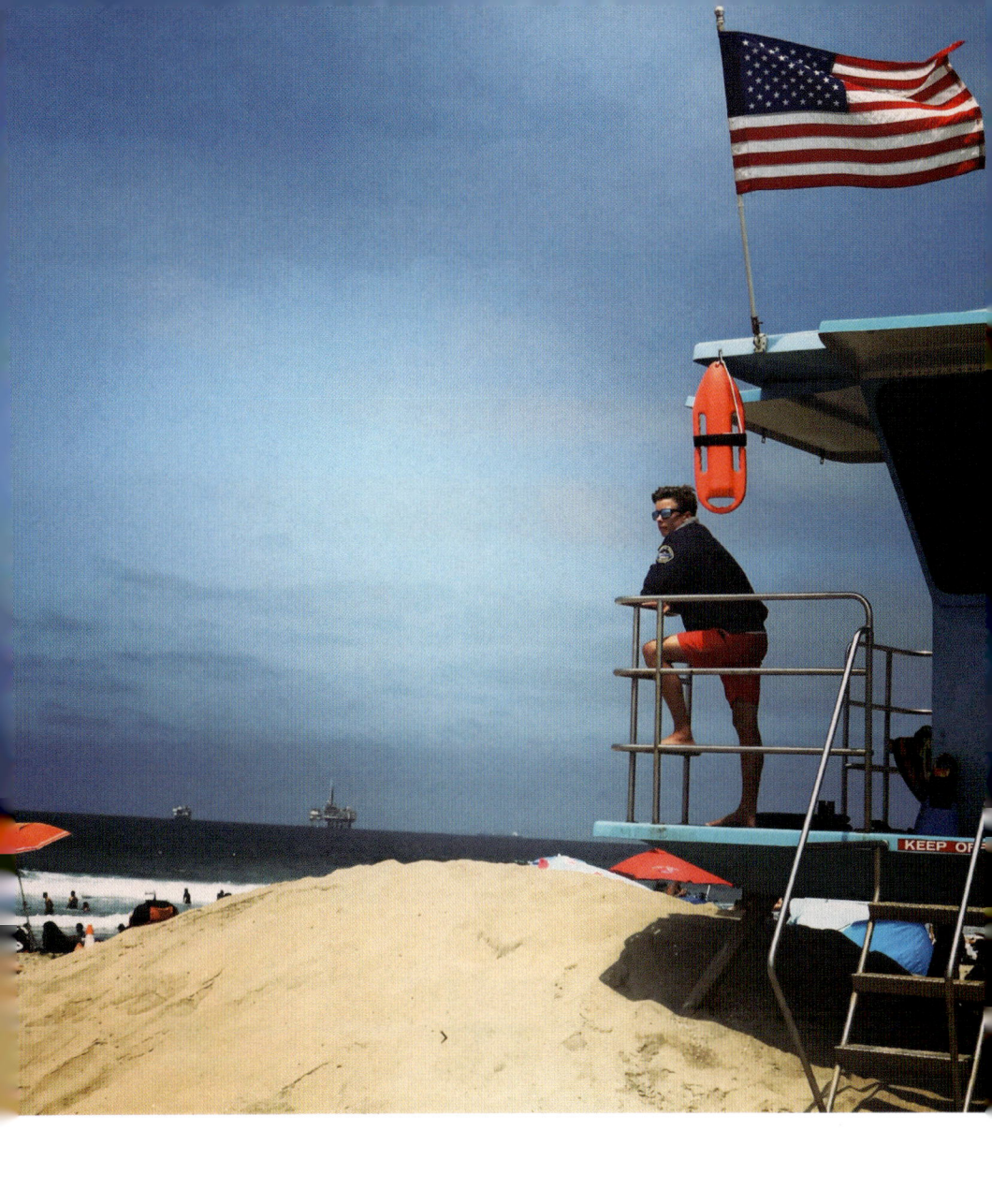

*"Tell me to what you pay attention and I will tell you who you are."*
~Jose Ortega

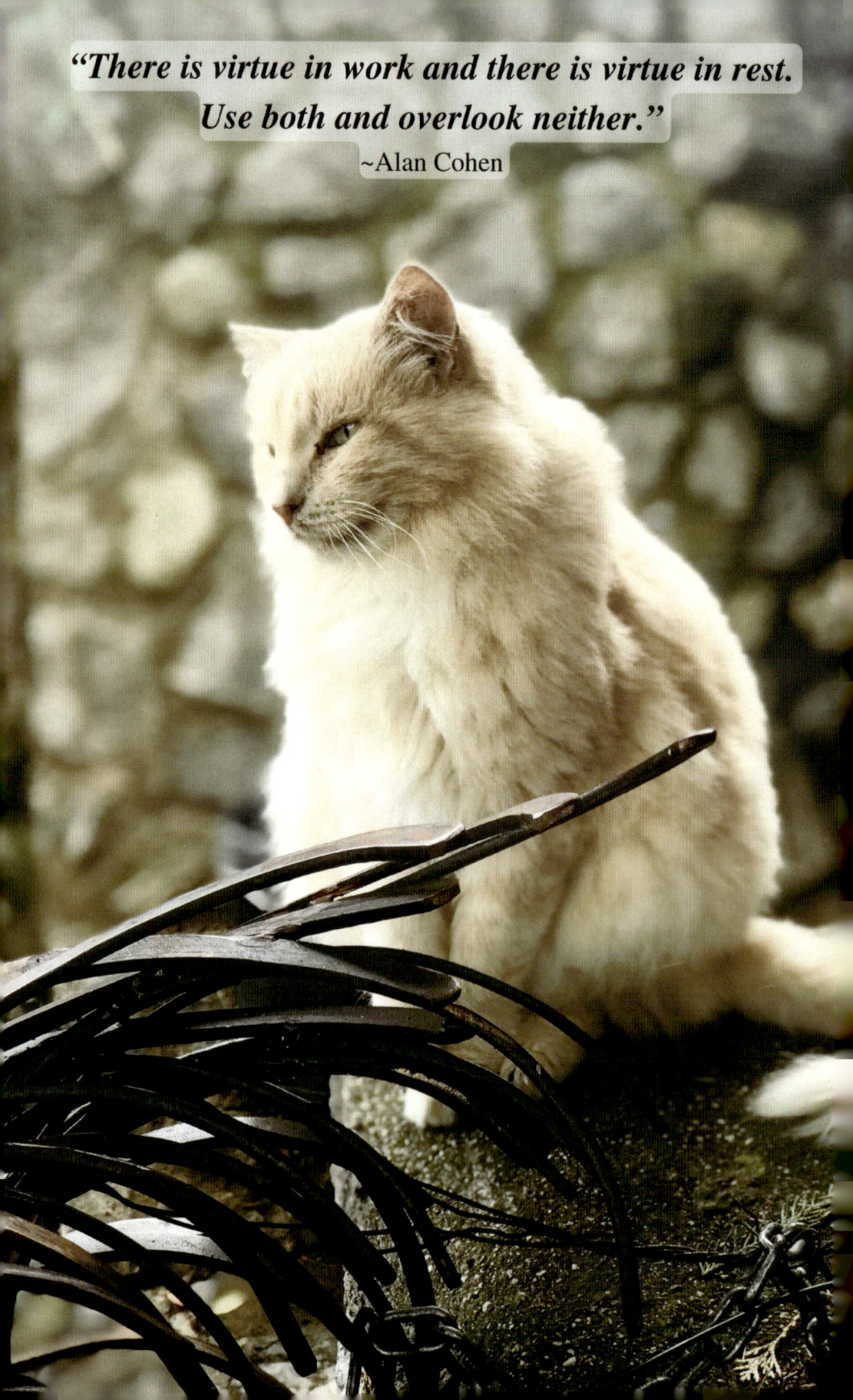

"There is virtue in work and there is virtue in rest.
Use both and overlook neither."
~Alan Cohen

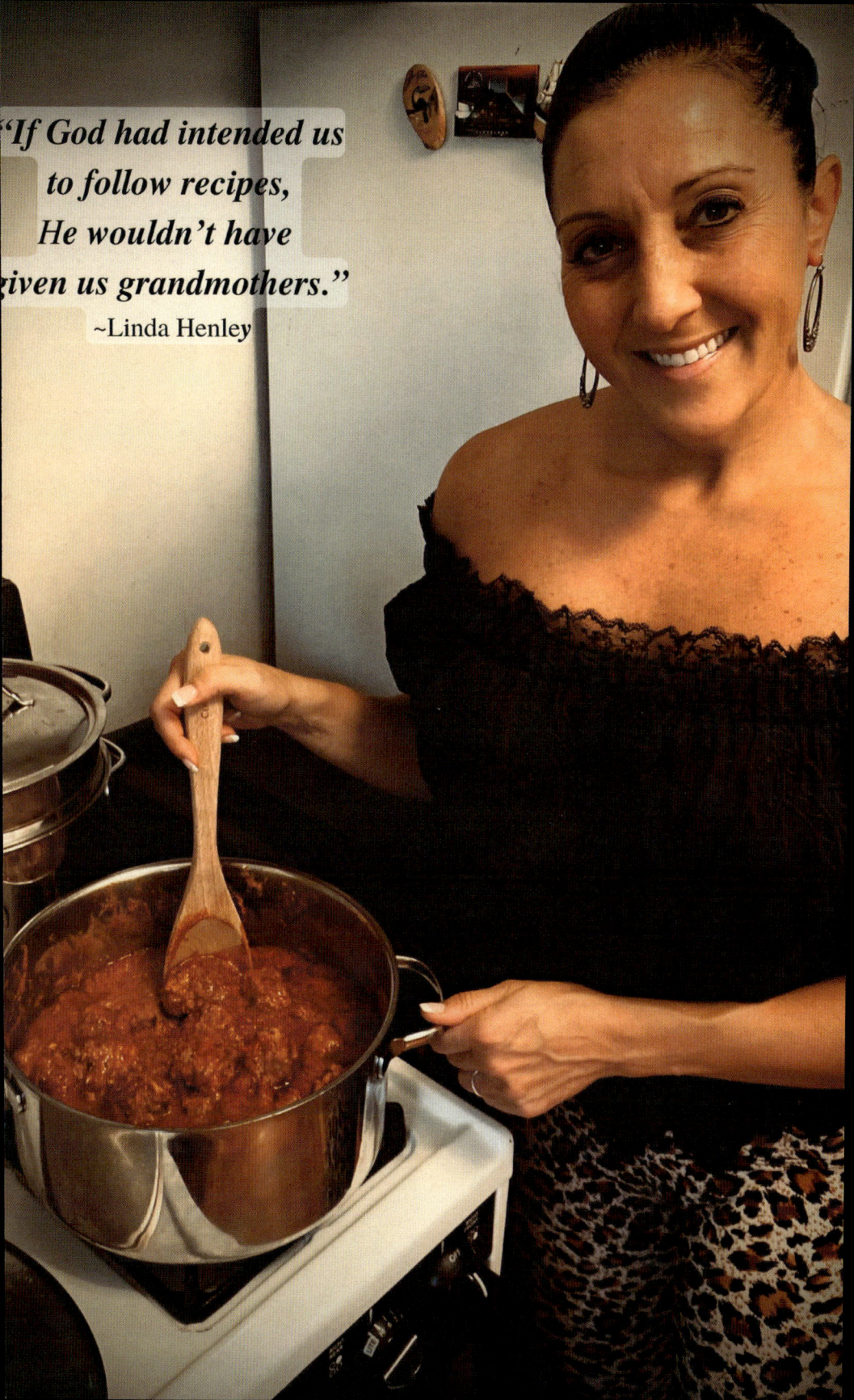

"If God had intended us to follow recipes, He wouldn't have given us grandmothers."
~Linda Henley

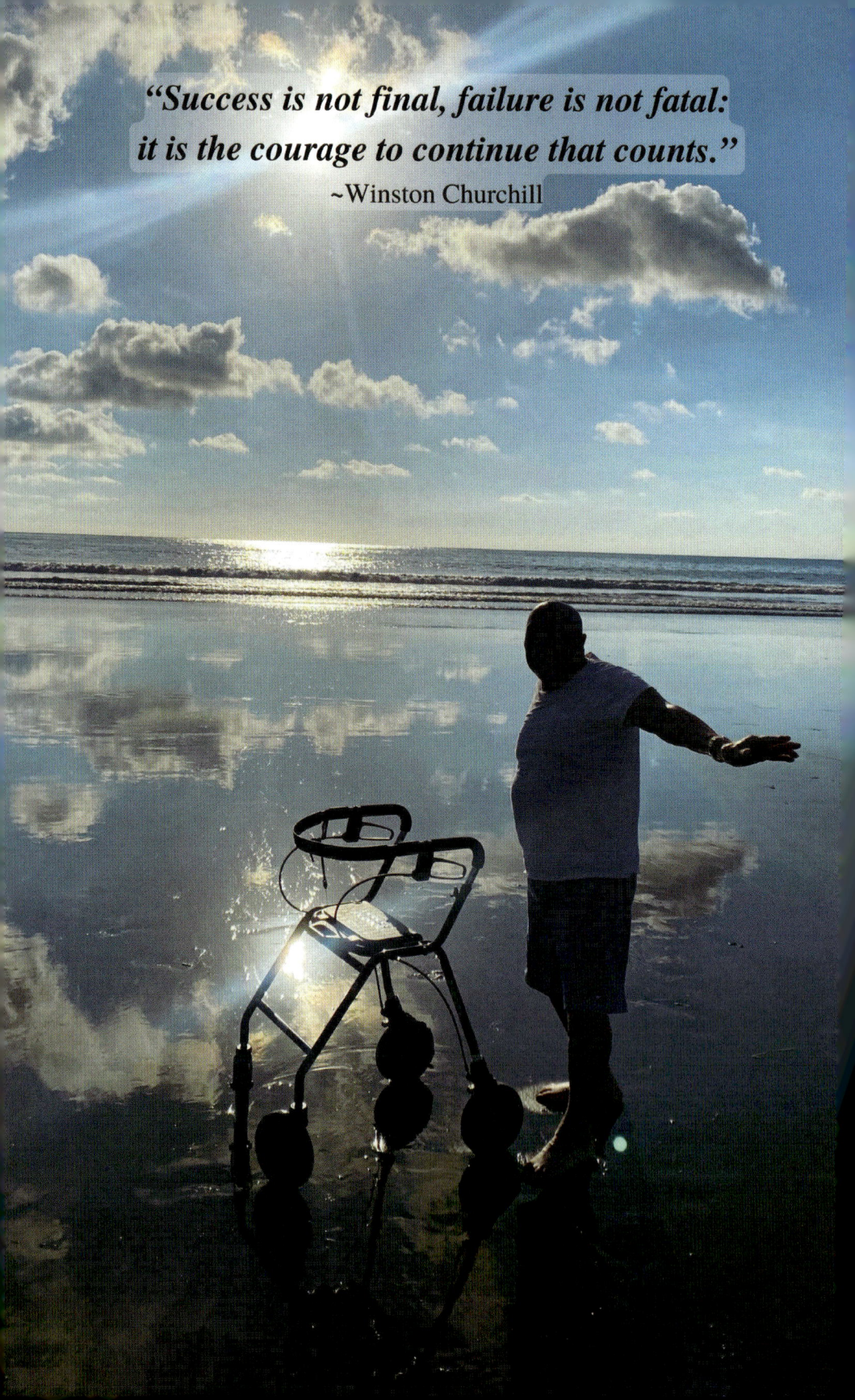

"Success is not final, failure is not fatal: it is the courage to continue that counts."
~Winston Churchill

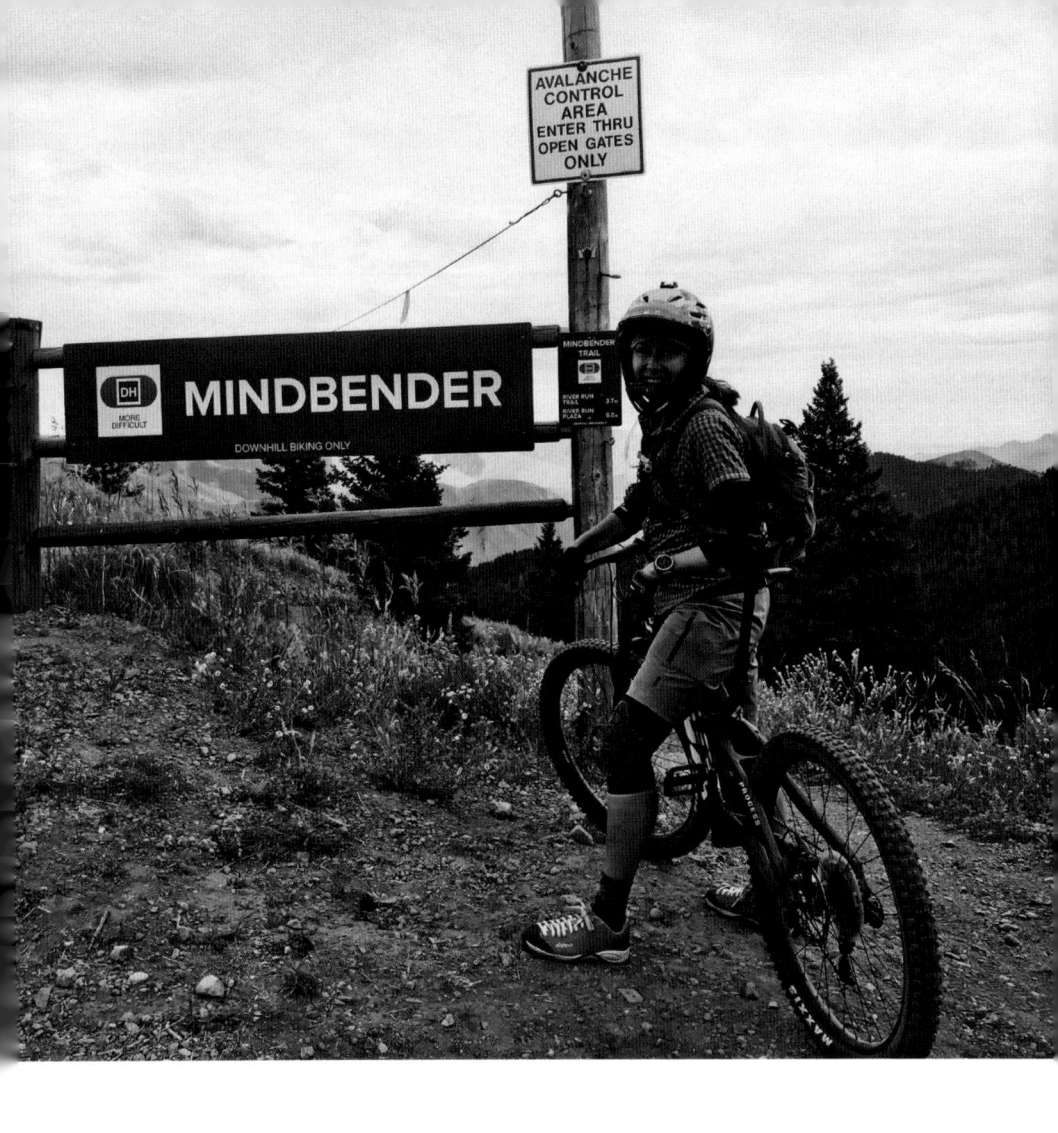

"By replacing fear of the unknown with curiosity we open ourselves up to an infinite stream of possibility. We can let fear rule our lives or we can become childlike with curiosity, pushing our boundaries, leaping out of our comfort zones, and accepting what life puts before us."

~Alan Watts

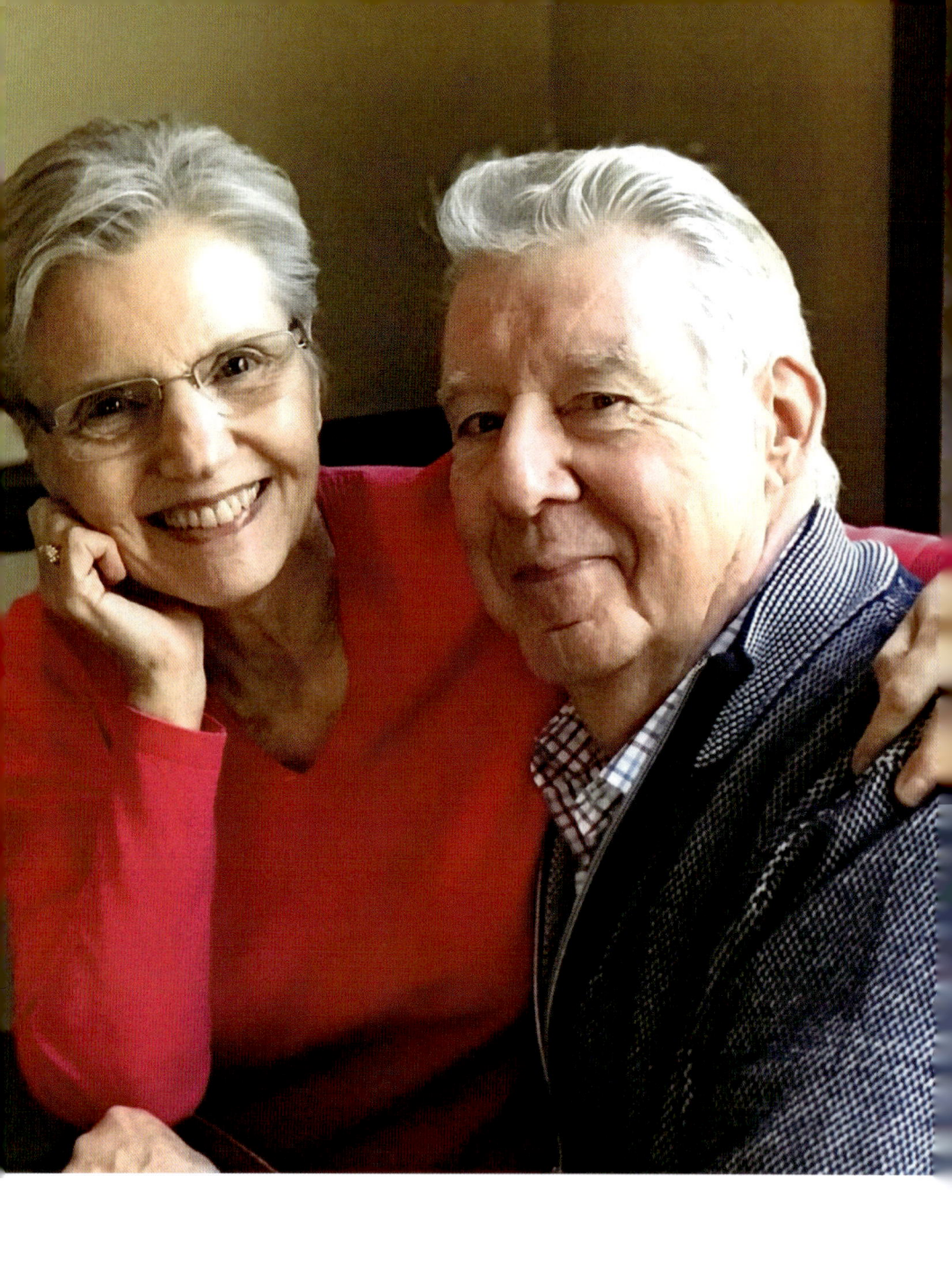

*"Let us always meet each other with a smile, for the smile is the beginning of love."*
~Mother Teresa

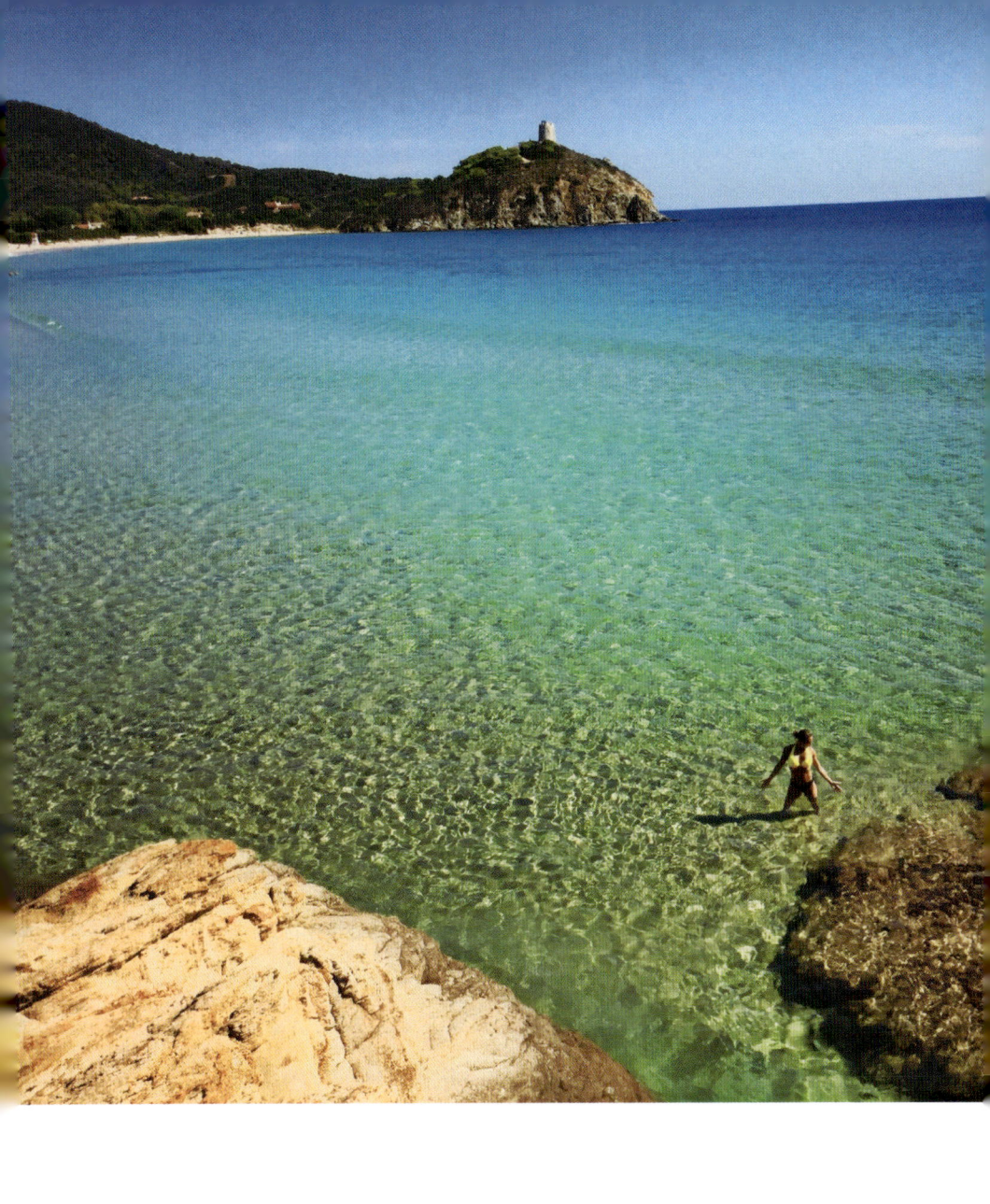

*have to be constantly reminded that the end goal of all of is striving is to live joyfully, and that there are often more direct ways of achieving this than conforming to rigid standards set by social customs."*
~Martha Beck

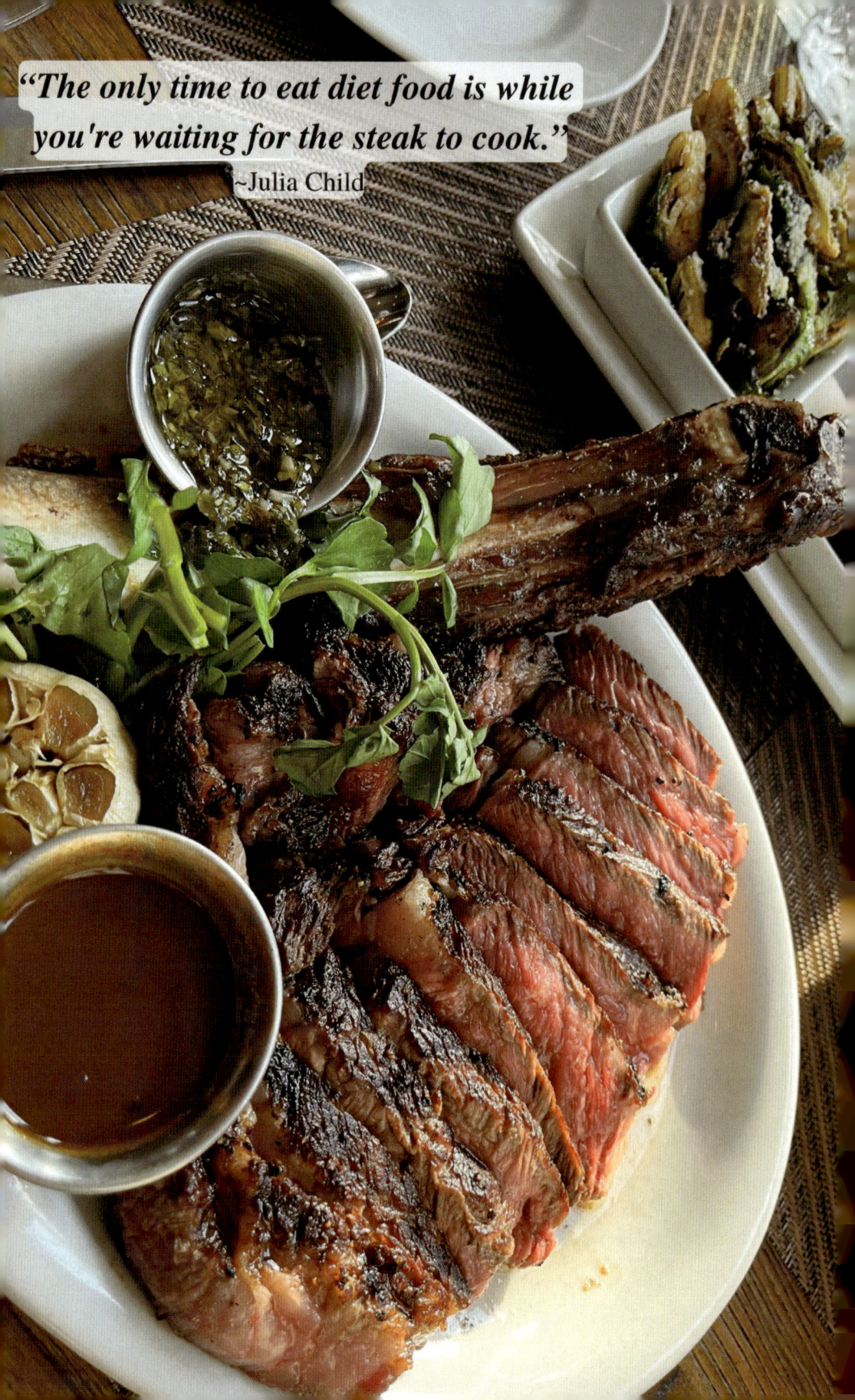

> "The only time to eat diet food is while you're waiting for the steak to cook."
> ~Julia Child

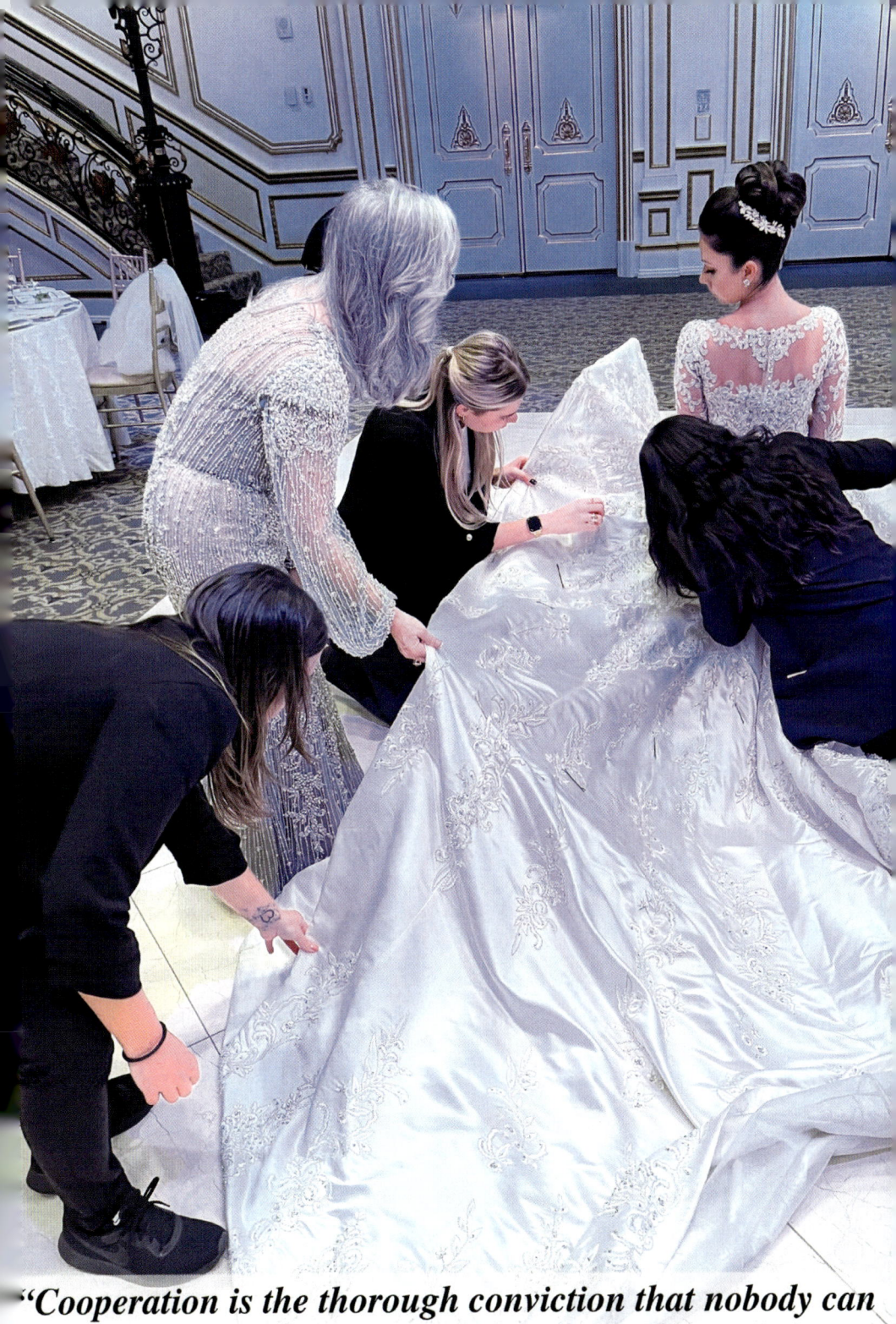

"Cooperation is the thorough conviction that nobody can get there unless everybody gets there."
~Virginia Burden

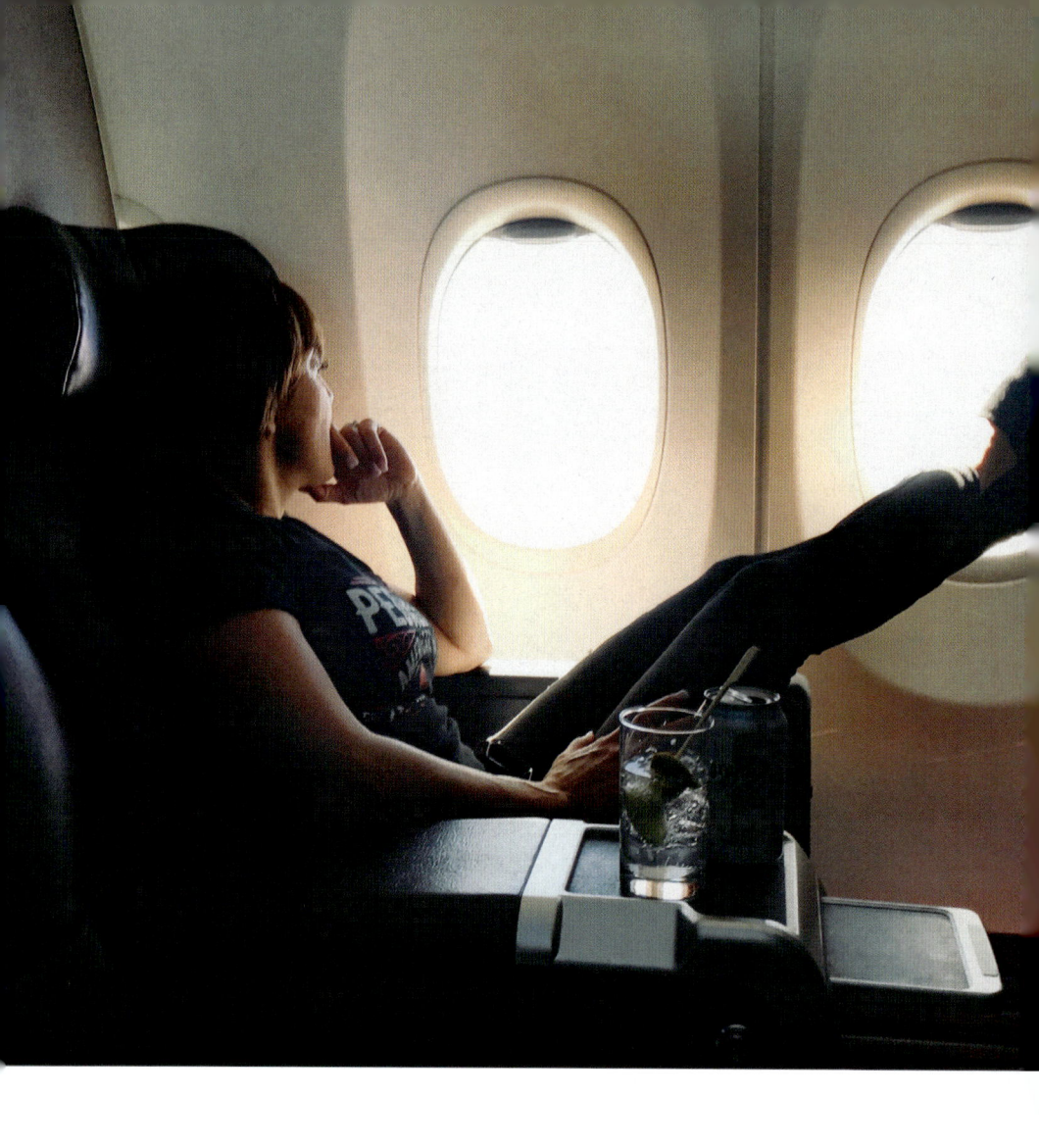

*"If the Universe has the wherewithal to inspire a desire within you, then it has the full capacity of gathering the components to make your desire a reality."*

~Abraham

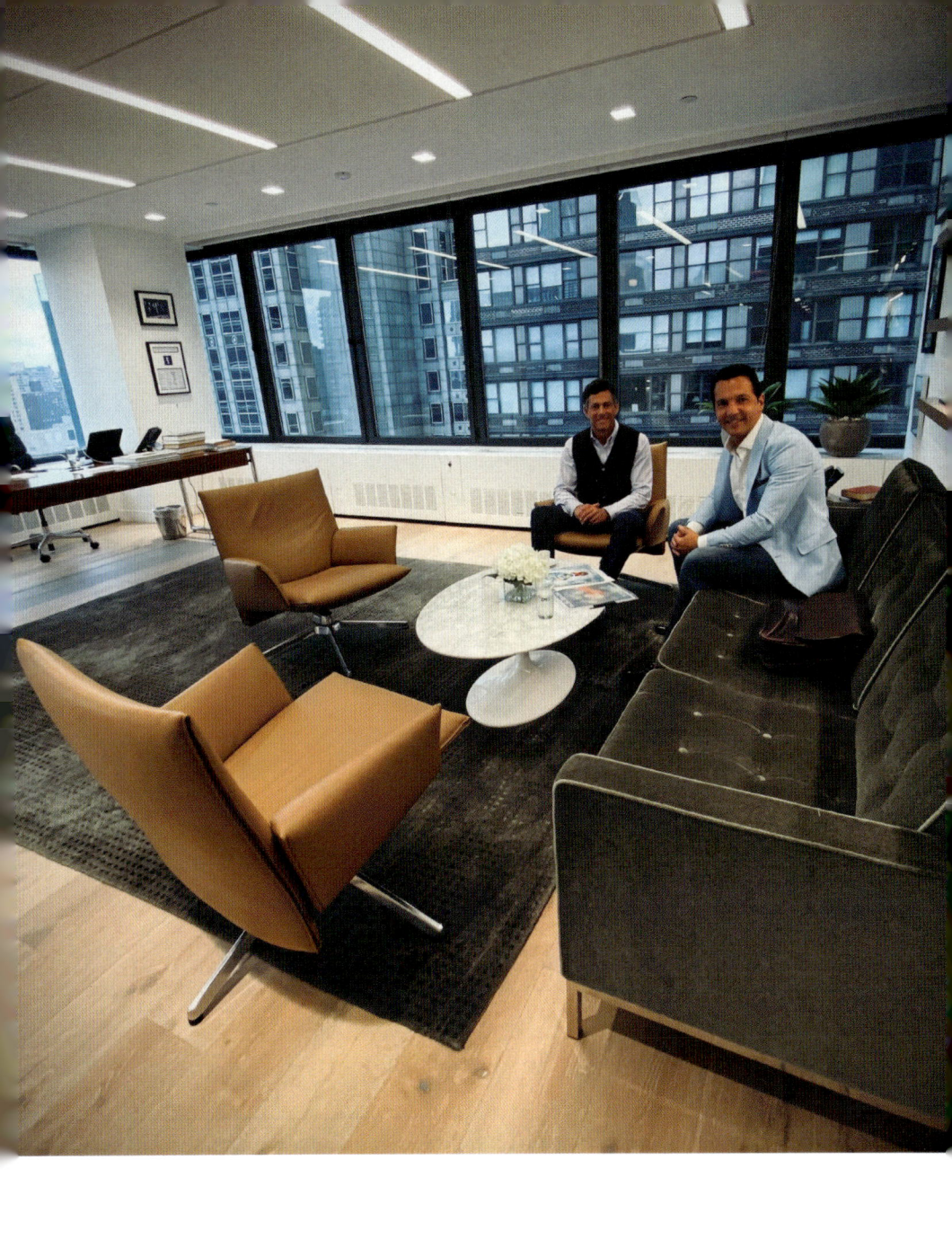

*"Education begins the gentleman, but reading, good company, and reflection must finish him."*
~John Locke

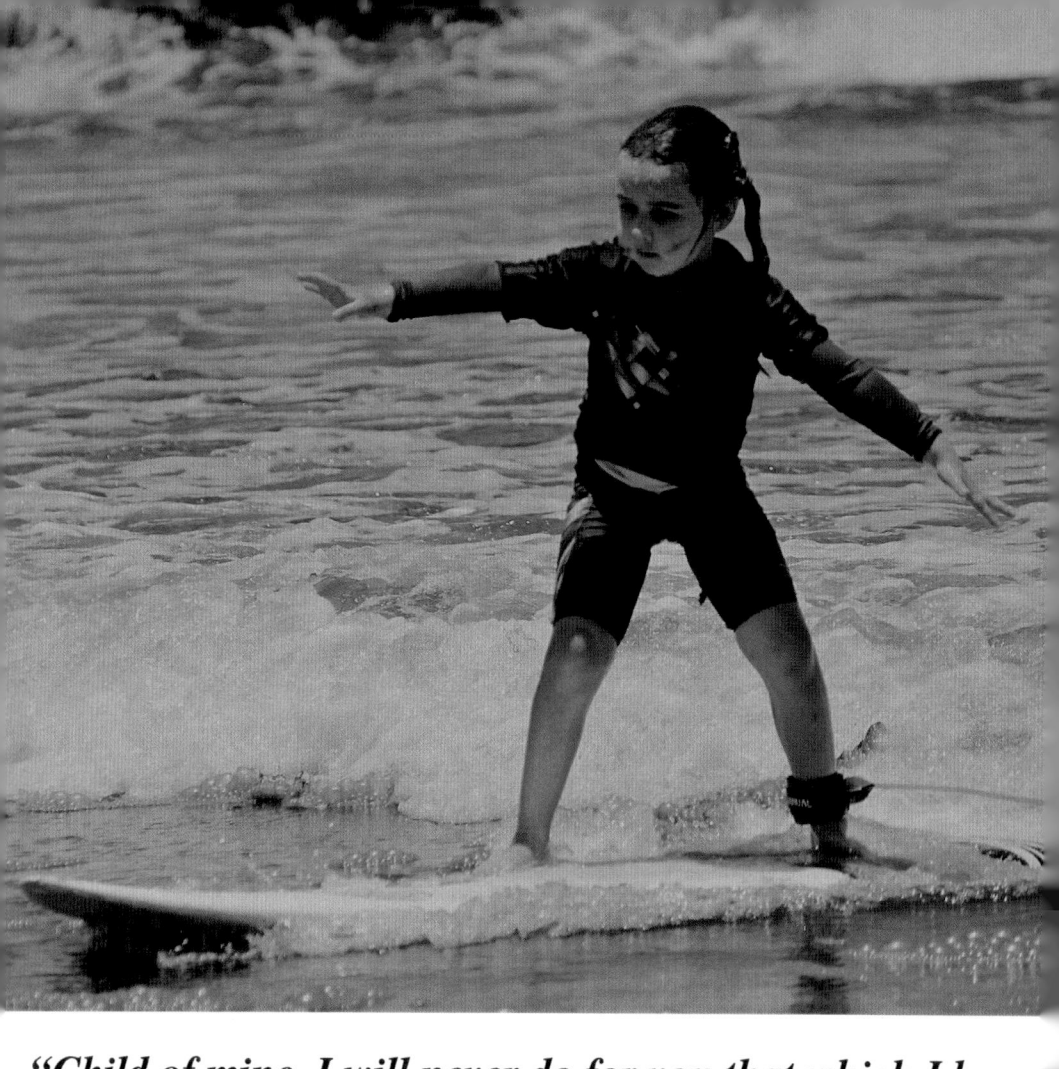

*"Child of mine, I will never do for you that which I know you can do for yourself. I will never rob you of an opportunity to show yourself your ability and talent. I will see you at all times as the capable, effective, powerful creator that you have come forth to be. And I will stand back as your most avid cheerleading section. But I will not do for you that which you have intended to do for yourself. Anything you need from me, ask. I'm always here to compliment or assist. I am here to encourage your growth, not justify my experience through you."*

~Abraham

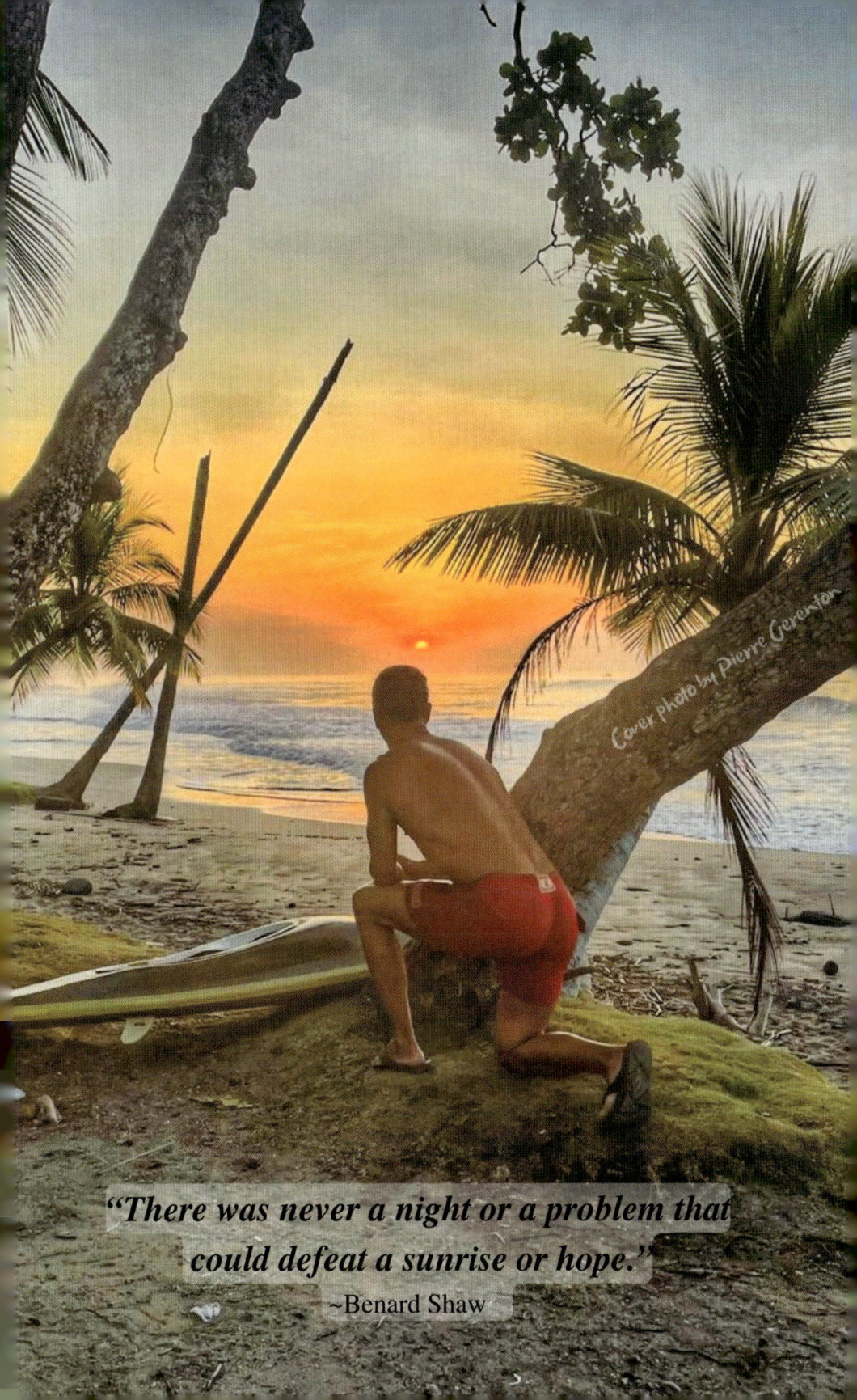

"There was never a night or a problem that could defeat a sunrise or hope."
~Benard Shaw

Cover photo by Pierre Gerenton

# RECOMMENDATION

**MY BLOG ON MARCELLOPEDALINO.COM** has a recurring book review feature called "Marcello Recommends." Each review article provides a comprehensive and detailed synopsis of the contents of the book and highlights some of my favorite excerpts. I found the books below to be educational, thought-provoking, relevant, humorous, worthwhile, or all of the above. I received a lot of positive feedback on the book recommendation list that I shared at the end of *Celebrate Life* so I'm hoping that you'll enjoy this *Onwards and Upwards* collection of new and noteworthy suggestions as well:

- Everyone Loves a Parade: *A Guide to New York City's Ticker Tape Parades* by Mark Walter and John Walter
- Golf Is Not a Game of Perfect by Dr. Bob Rotella
- The Plus: *Self-Help for People Who Hate Self-Help* by Greg Gutfeld
- I Love It Here: *How Great Leaders Create Organizations Their People Never Want to Leave* by Clint Pulver
- Top Visionaries Who Changed the World by George Ilian
- Becoming Ageless: *The Four Secrets to Looking and Feeling Younger Than Ever* by Strauss Zelnick
- Attention Pays: *How to Drive Profitability*, Productivity, and Accountability by Neen James
- Waiting For The Punch: *Words to Live by* from the WTF Podcast by Marc Maron
- On This Date In Music: *A Day to Day History of the Music that Inspires Us and the Artists Who Create It* by Mike Walter
- The Blue Zones of Happiness: *A Blueprint for a Better Life* by Dan Buettner

# APPRECIATION

**I WOULD LIKE TO EXTEND** a special thank you to everyone who played a meaningful role in helping me complete my second book, and officially become "an author." I know your time and energy are precious, so please know that I appreciate you.

- Dr. Jill Pedalino
- Mike Walter
- Neen James
- Randy Bartlett
- Pierre Gerenton
- Dave Kotinsky
- Strauss Zelnick
- Dan Buettner

…and to my miracle matchmaker, Jaime, for setting Jill and me up on a blind date and making that fateful three-hour cup of tea possible.

# CONNECTION

**IF YOU WOULD LIKE ADDITIONAL** assistance moving onwards and upwards via a private consultation, keynote speaking engagement, media appearance, or upcoming event for the organization you represent, please call or text 732-547-1677 or visit MarcelloPedalino.com for booking information and further details.

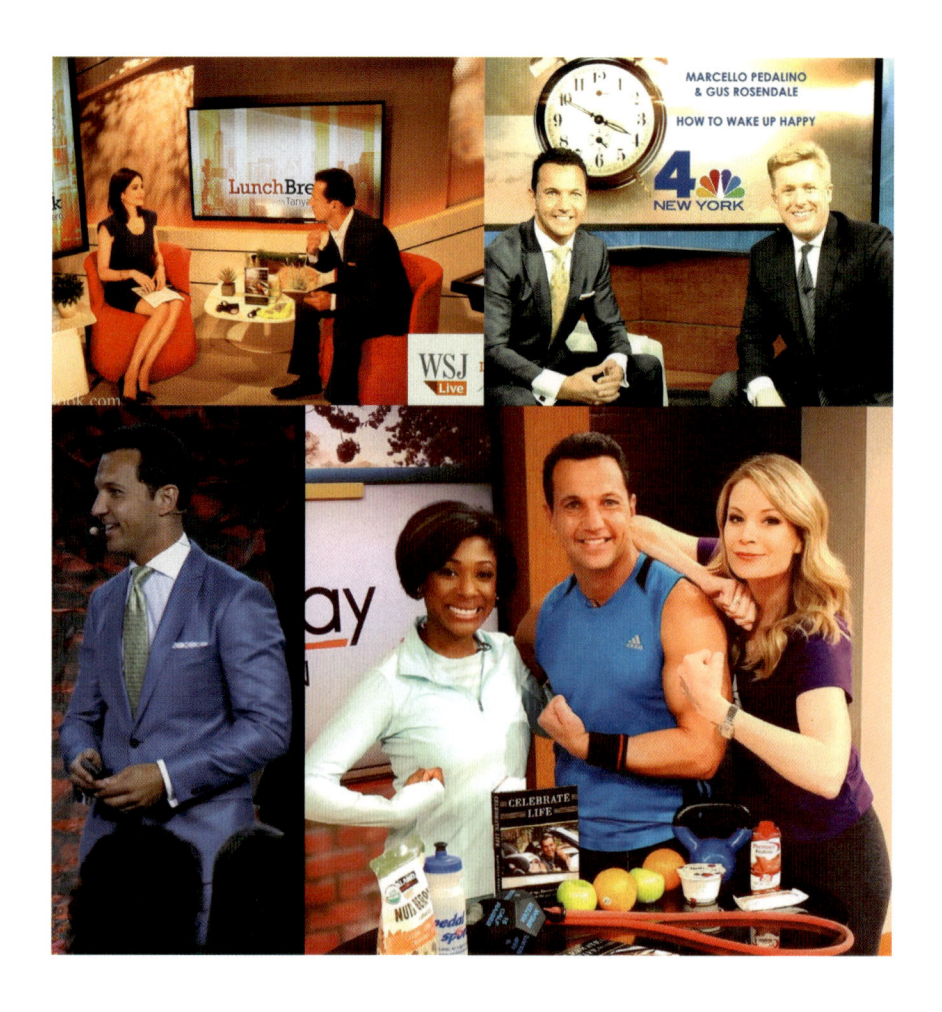

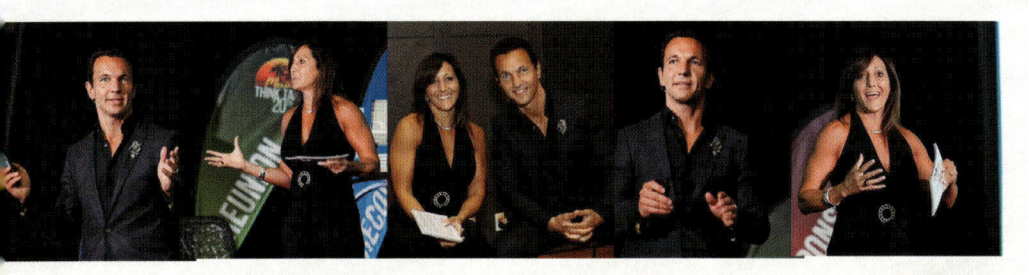

"...arcello and Dr. Jill are masters of both 'talking the talk' and 'walking ...e walk'. **Their unique life experiences and perspective offers ...udiences an opportunity to shift their mindset, habits, and ultimately, their own future."**
-David Osbourne, Georgia

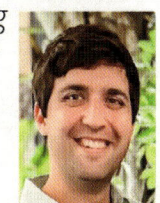

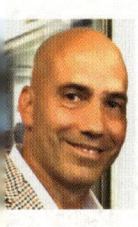

"What an awesome way to kick off the week! **I knew when Dr. Jill and Marcello started their presentation this was going to be an amazing conference.**" -Robert Arthur, California

"Based on their 'Solutions Create Momentum' philosophy, **I hit the ground running as soon as I left the conference!**"
-Kristin Wilson, Florida

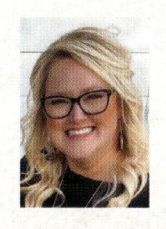

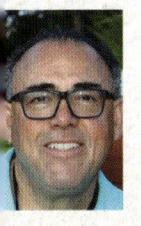

"Dr. Jill and Marcello's keynote, Onwards and Upwards, really spoke to me. Specifically, these three things: **Success comes with a price...and the currency is time, Change your environment, change your life, and Define my 'Tribe of Influence'...Who are the people I want to start spending more time with?** Thank you both for sharing your special wisdom and experience to truly impact our lives." -Jorge Lopez, California

"I really enjoyed the Onwards and Upwards presentation. It's very ...ch in line with my philosophy and values, and **it's always great to ...challenged to ask, 'I know this, but how well am I living it?'**"
-Miles Gilbert, Arizona

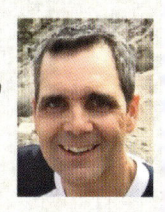

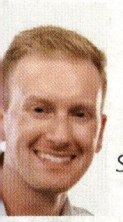

"Thank you for delivering such a powerful keynote to our group. **I believe it was one of the most impactful sessions of the symposium**. I heard over and over again during our 'takeaways' segment on the last day people recounting parts of your presentation."
-David Meister, Florida

# WORKS CITED

Buettner, Dan. *The Blue Zones of Happiness*: A Blueprint for a Better Life. National Geographic, 2017.

"Good Thing Bad Thing Who Knows - TheGentlemanPhilsopher.com" The Gentleman Philosopher Blog 10 May 2023. 24 Feb. 2023.

"How to deal with failure and bad situations. - Youtube.com" The Jocko Podcast 25 Jan. 2015. 24 Feb. 2023 https://www.youtube.com/watch?v=IdTMDpizis8/

Sansone-Braff, Cindi. *Grant Me A Higher Love*: How to Go from the Relationship from Hell to One that's Heaven Sent by Scaling The Ladder of Love. Book Surge, 2008.

"Strong Convictions Loosely Held - PeterAttiaMd.com" Peter Attia Md Blog 6 April 2020. 24 Feb. 2023. https://peterattiamd.com/strong-convictions-loosely-held/

"The Missing Sugar Bowl - Reddit.com " Jokes Page. 24 Feb 2023. https://www.reddit.com/r/Jokes/comments/nnlqqu/the_missing_sugar_bowl/

"The Story of the Mexican Fisherman - BeMoreWithLess.com." Be More With Less Home Page. 24 Feb. 2023. https://bemorewithless.com/the-story-of-the-mexican-fisherman/

"Watch Your Thoughts - GoodReads.com" Good Reads Quotable Quotes Page Lao Tzu. 24 Feb. 2023 https://www.goodreads.com/quotes/8203490-watch-your-thoughts-they-become-your-words-watch-your-words/

# ABOUT THE AUTHOR

**MARCELLO PEDALINO, CFT, CNC, CLC,** is a lifestyle expert. As a certified fitness trainer, nutrition consultant, and lifespan coach, he delivers meaningful keynote presentations that help people prioritize work-life integration and recognize the importance of energy management. Marcello is the author of Celebrate Life: How to live it up, discover fulfillment, and experience the joy you deserve. He loves being the class Dad for his daughter, being the CEO of his wife's medical practice, and of course— helping the world Celebrate Life with his entertainment and event production company.

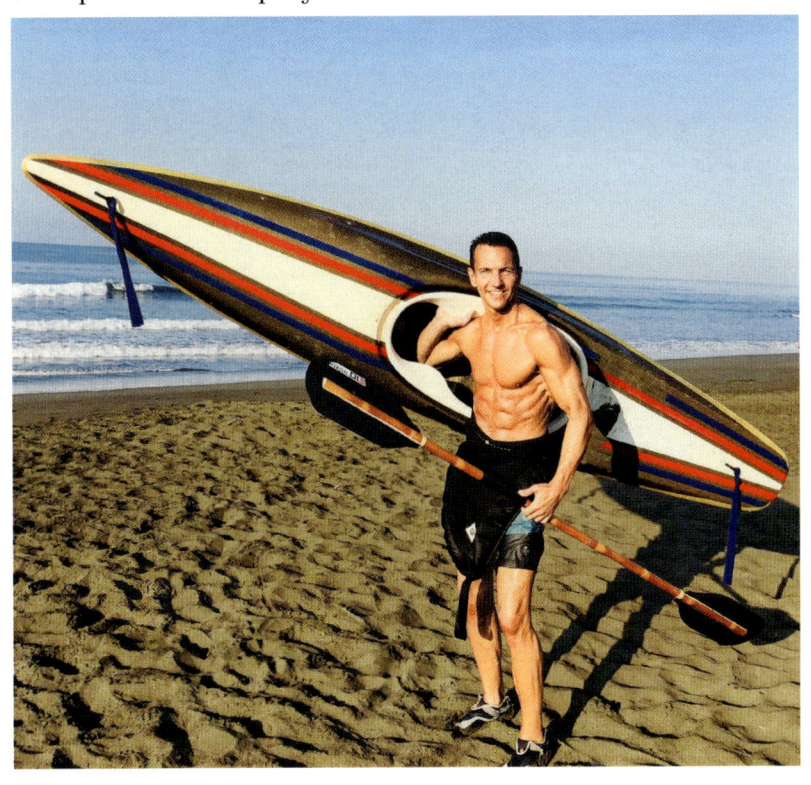

# P.S.

Isabella,

If I'm still around ten years from now, maybe I'll keep up the tradition and you'll get another book of life lessons to add to your collection. Until then, I hope you continue to celebrate life every day. Always find something to smile about and be grateful for when we ask you, "What was your favorite part of the day?" at bedtime. Laugh a lot, be kind, remember that family comes first, order your steak medium rare, and keep on starting your mornings by singing *Defying Gravity* from *Wicked* at the top of your lungs. Onwards and Upwards!

> "It's time to try defying gravity, and you can't pull me down!"

Love,<br>
Daddy